Juicing Cannabis for Healing

How I Achieved Almost Complete Remission of Chronic Pain by Juicing Fresh Raw Marijuana Leaf

by

Katie Marsh

Copyright © 2015 Katie Marsh
First Paperbound Printing
Printed in the USA

All rights reserved. No part of this book may be reproduced in any form or transmitted by any means – electronic, mechanical, or otherwise – including photography, recording, or any information storage and retrieval system, without permission in writing from the author.

Cover design by Fiverr Creator
Edited by Edmund Weisberg, MS, MBE
Fifth Dimension Press

Table of Contents

- **CHAPTER 1**
  - INTRODUCTION 5
- **CHAPTER 2**
  - WHY JUICE IT? 8
- **CHAPTER 3**
  - THE BACK STORY 12
- **CHAPTER 4**
  - WHY I WROTE THIS BOOK 14
- **CHAPTER 5**
  - SOME OF THE DISEASES CANNABIS JUICE HELPS ALLEVIATE AND/OR PUT INTO A SUSTAINED REMISSION 31
- **CHAPTER 6**
  - HOW CANNABINOIDS WORK 39
- **CHAPTER 7**
  - SUGGESTED DOSAGE 45
- **CHAPTER 8**
  - WHERE TO GET THE JUICE 51
- **CHAPTER 9**
  - JUICING TIPS 60
- **CHAPTER 10**
  - CANNABIS OIL, TINCTURE & SALVE 68
- **CHAPTER 11**
  - TESTIMONIALS 78
- **APPENDIX A**
  - LINKS TO US STATES' LAWS REGARDING MEDICAL MARIJUANA 88
- **APPENDIX B**
  - LIST OF SEED BANKS 93
- **APPENDIX C**
  - US STATES ALLOWED TO GROW HEMP FOR RESEARCH AS PER 2014 US FARM BILL 96
- **APPENDIX D**
  - LINKS TO US CONGRESS LISTED BY STATE AND DISTRICT 106
- OTHER BOOKS BY KATIE MARSH 110

"Education is the most powerful weapon which you can use to change the world."

— Nelson Mandela

"Herb is the healing of a nation, alcohol is the destruction."

— Bob Marley

"They always say time changes things, but you actually have to change them yourself."

— Andy Warhol

Chapter 1
Introduction

As I started to write this book, I went to my usual coffee house to conduct research using their free WiFi. But access to the websites I needed was blocked from view; the message on the screen was "Inappropriate Content." I'm not sure exactly what is inappropriate about the most healing plant on earth.

I am not a medical professional, scientist, or cannabis research expert. I'm just someone who needed a solution to an illness and found it in this natural herb. This book is intended for those afflicted with various chronic conditions, or acute symptoms, who have tried all manner of legal pharmaceutical and natural remedies without success. Please consult with your medical doctor, holistic health practitioner, guru and/or your higher self to see if this treatment is right for you. And above all else **go slowly** with the dosing. Each individual is different; every disease has its nuances. If you are not growing the plant yourself, you may not know if the THC (tetrahydrocannabinol), one of the key active ingredients in cannabis, has been activated inadvertently due to touching a grow light or becoming heated during transport. If a plant is grown outdoors in very hot weather, occasionally the top of the plant may become psychoactive but this is rare. But if the plant has not been heated, you should not experience any high feeling at all. But remember: If you didn't grow it, you don't know it.

For certain medical conditions, it is not advisable to juice cannabis, unless your medical professional tells you otherwise. For example, a cannabis juicing regimen is not recommended if you have kidney or gallbladder problems, hypercalciuria (also known as hypercalcinuria), or hyperoxaluria. And anyone taking prescription medications that can be blocked by pomegranate or grapefruit should talk to their doctor first. Also, individuals taking blood-thinning medications such as Coumadin should probably not juice cannabis unless advised by their medical professional first (http://www.alternet.org/personal-health/juicing-raw-cannabis-miracle-health-cure-some-its-proponents-believe-it-be).

The information presented in this book may or may not comply with your local state law or even federal law. I am not offering any legal or medical advice whatsoever, just information that I have been able to obtain through research, consultations, phone calls, and my personal experience. As I learn more, I will update this eBook and the hard copy on Amazon. If you wish to receive the latest updates without having to repurchase this book each time, please sign up for my mailing list at juicingcannabisforhealing.com.

Lastly, if you are the type of person who wants a quick and easy fix—some pill you can purchase from your local pharmacy—then this book is definitely not for you. It's a relatively quick fix, with most people seeing results in a month or sooner but, at this time, it's far from easy to obtain. If, like me, you are desperate enough to try anything and persistent enough to seek what you need, then please read on.

Chapter 2
Why Juice It?

It's simple. Heating the bud destroys many of the beneficial healing compounds in the plant but juicing it allows you to receive all the benefits of the healing molecules in perfect balanced synergy. Juicing is especially healing for people with compromised immune systems and for anyone who needs a powerful anti-inflammatory agent. In my experience it works much better than turmeric, drinking fresh ginger tea all day, and even better than popping Motrin like candy.

Some people don't like inhaling carbon into their lungs; therefore, smoking it isn't a preferable option for pain relief. So there are vaporizing devices on the market as an alternative option. Ideally the vaporizer heats up the dried bud to 446 degrees F, which is considered the point where the most of the CBG cannabinoid is released. It is also the point where most all the THCa is converted to THC (http://www.hightimes.com/read/studying-vaporizer-insight-proper-vape-use). More about cannabinoids later in Chapter 6, How Cannabinoids Work.

Smoking of the bud heats it above approximately 554 F, which is the point where tar and carcinogens are released from the plant. Vaporized cannabis contains water along with THC (tetrahydrocannabinol), the cannabinoid in cannabis that offers pain relief and the "high" feeling. Vaporizing allows the user to inhale THC without inhaling the carbon from burning the plant and smoking it.

I've never personally tried these but, according to my medical marijuana doctor, two of the best and most affordable vaporizers on the market are the Vapor Genie and the Solo. The Solo is more expensive than the Vapor Genie but it's supposed to be easier to control than the Vapor Genie and it hides the odor of the cannabis well so that no one knows your business.

When you use a vaporizer, do not light it with a lighter. It's not a great idea to inhale butane. Instead, light a match, wait a moment for the sulfur to burn off and then light the cannabis according to the manufacturer's directions.

One other little trick about vaporizers: When you're using a vaporizer like the Solo, take a pen cap and put it into the mouthpiece when you are not inhaling. This will help to keep the vapor in the tube so that it does not get wasted by escaping. And you will know you are vaporizing correctly when, upon exhale, you can taste the cannabis and you can see a bit of vapor escape but no smoke.

If or when you need to drive a vehicle and you have your cannabis and/or paraphernalia with you, make sure you purchase a case that you can lock. Put it in the case, set it in your backseat and refrain from reaching for or opening it unless you are asked to by law enforcement. Also carry your medical marijuana card with you. In the event that you get pulled over, it will be obvious to law enforcement that you were not smoking or vaporizing while driving. This is just a little tip to keep all of us safe and out of trouble with law enforcement officials. Of course, it is well known that driving under the influence of alcohol is much more dangerous than operating a vehicle after having used marijuana.

Although vaporizing is better for your lungs than smoking, juicing cannabis leaf and bud is the superior way to receive all of the healing benefits of this amazing plant. Just as many raw food advocates claim that when you cook a food above 108 F you kill many of the beneficial vitamins and enzymes, when you heat cannabis bud to smoke it you are killing many of the beneficial cannabinoids. There are 80 known cannabinoids found in the plant so far. Incidentally, some cannabinoids can also be found in Echinacea.

CBD or cannabidiol (pronounced ca nab eu **die** ol) is thought to be the most important molecule in the plant. When the plant is not heated but consumed in its raw form, THC and CBD are not activated. Rather, the molecules that are consumed are THCa (THC acid) and CBDa (CBD acid.) In acid form, CBD is the most healing and beneficial constituent to your body and THC, in acid form, will not get you high. It is the *heating* of the plant—any part of the plant whether it's the leaf or the bud—that decarboxylates the CBDa and THCa, turning it into CBD and THC. And, as you know, THC will get you high. For more information about the decarboxylation process, please see: http://bit.ly/1tig0Le.

This book is about how to juice the plant to receive all the healing benefits of CBDa and the other cannabinoids. Please see Chapter 5, Some of the Diseases Cannabis Juice Helps Alleviate and/or Put into a Sustained Remission for extensive information about all of the health benefits of cannabinoids.

The cannabis plant is believed to have been in existence for over 34 million years. It is thought that animals and humans have grazed on this plant to receive its healing benefits throughout history. As humans learned to cultivate and manipulate the genetics of the plant, the amount of THCa it contains has greatly increased, thus lowering the amount of CBDa due to the inverse relationship between THCa and CBDa. In other words, the higher the amount of THCa, the lower the CBDa; the lower the THCa level in the plant the higher the amount of CBDa.

In recent years we have learned that we can consume greater quantities of fruits, vegetables, and grasses (such as wheatgrass) by processing the plants through a juicing machine. The only disadvantage is that you don't get to consume as much of the plant fiber when juicing. But if you did eat it, you would be so full that you wouldn't be able to take as much of the plant into your body anyway.

Chapter 3
The Back Story

Kristen Courtney and her husband, William Courtney, MD, are pioneers in the field of dietary cannabis. Kristen suffered through several diseases as a teen and young adult. She was bedridden with autoimmune disorders such as rheumatoid arthritis (RA) and lupus. As a young adult, she was taking over 40 medications and told that due to her severe endometriosis she would never be able to bear children. At one point she started smoking and ingesting a significant quantity of marijuana, soon noticing that besides helping her manage her pain the herb helped reduce the number of infections she experienced. So she moved from a state that prohibits medical marijuana to California in order to grow her own medicine. Please watch her video at http://bit.ly/WqK38X.

When Kristen moved to Northern California, she met Dr. Courtney and eventually they married and had several children. When he first started counseling patients about medical cannabis, he advised them to consume capsules of dried cannabis leaf. Later he discovered that juicing the raw plant leaves and buds yielded the greatest medical benefits.

So Kristen started juicing any leaf she could obtain. At the time, there were no labs available to the public to test for THCa and

CBDa content of cannabis strains. So she tried to select leaf that was purplish in color because those strains were believed to contain the highest amount of CBDa, the most valuable cannabinoid in marijuana. Kristen was juicing about 8 ounces a day and after a month she was able to wean herself from most of her 40 medications and start to live a normal life. She became fully healed over time and continues to juice to this day.

The rare times in her life when she has been unable to access fresh leaf for juicing, her various disease symptoms began to return. As soon as she was able to begin juicing again, they subsided. She believes that she has clinical endocannabinoid deficiency (CECD) syndrome that is the root cause of her symptoms and various diagnosed diseases. Drinking raw cannabis juice provides the missing cannabinoids that her body needs. Kristen even juiced cannabis during her pregnancies. Her doctors, for political reasons, would not tell her to consume cannabis during pregnancy. But they did recommend that she continue doing whatever it was she was doing to remain healthy. Again, this was a woman who was told she would never bear children due to her severe endometriosis.

What struck me most about the Courtneys' video was their sincerity. Also striking was how sick Kristen had been yet how beautiful and healthy she appeared to be in the video. All I had was RA and here was a woman who had RA, lupus, and numerous other disorders. Doctors had given up hope of her leading a normal life and they were just trying to keep her comfortable in her bedridden state. I felt compelled to learn more.

Chapter 4
Why I Wrote This Book

I was officially diagnosed with RA near the beginning of 2012, but I have been suffering with the symptoms of this autoimmune condition since 2009. As with many diseases, this one has proved to be progressive in nature. At my worst, I could barely get dressed, hold a fork, open a package or bottle, sit down or stand up, or walk across the floor, up stairs, or down the block. This was a far cry from my early 20s when I competed in Ironman triathlons, Escape from Alcatraz triathlons, and marathons just for fun and to challenge myself. RA was proving to be the greatest challenge of my life.

After consulting with many in the natural health community, I have tried probably every natural remedy on the market to no avail. I also experimented with dietary changes. I went on a strict gluten-free diet for two months with no results. I went on a five-day juice fast. Nothing. I went paleo for a month. No results except a flatter tummy. I did the elimination diet. Zero help for me. The funny thing is that dietary changes back then didn't help me at all yet eating the wrong foods today (sugar, pork), after experiencing healing from juicing, can hurt me. And doing yoga and managing my stress always helps.

Anyway, not being one to immediately turn to pharmaceuticals to treat or mask my symptoms without addressing underlying causes, I searched for a natural cure. One day while playing at a local park with my kids a friend told me about the Courtneys and their video.

Marijuana has been in the mainstream news most days lately. Whether it is for medical purposes or recreational, it seems our social mores are changing with regard to this ancient healing plant. But little is known about how to obtain the greatest health benefits of all from cannabis—consuming the plant in its raw form.

After watching the video, I called to make an appointment to see Dr. William Courtney in Northern California. He's a very busy physician so it took me a couple of months to get an appointment.

When meeting with Dr. Courtney, he presented a new option that didn't appear in his videos. There was a strain of cannabis called ACDC 22:1. ACDC stands for "Alternative Cannabinoid Dietary Cannabis," meaning that it contains 22 parts CBD to 1 part THC. He said I should try to obtain this plant because it contains the most CBD of any cannabis plant. When I asked him where I could get it, he said he was not able to tell me this because technically, as a doctor, this would be considered "aiding and abetting." But he suggested that I call around to some local dispensaries and maybe I would find it.

After the appointment I made a couple of calls and sure enough found that Herban Legend (http://bit.ly/1rzgTP5) dispensary in nearby Fort Bragg, California, carried the ACDC 22:1 clones. They never seem to have any seeds, though, only clones.

According to www.growweedeasy.com, a clone is "a little piece of plant that has been cut off from a parent plant and then given the opportunity to root on its own. You will want to take clones off a cannabis plant when it's in the vegetative stage, and you will tend to get better results if you use clones from a well-established plant (at least two months old). If you grow a plant in the vegetative stage for about 2-3 months, you will be able to get dozens of clones off it.

"Each cannabis clone is a genetic copy of its parent, so if the parent is a female, then you are guaranteed that all the clones taken from that cannabis plant will be female. This can be a great way of propagating a cannabis strain without having to ever worry about male plants or seeds. Each clone is also completely mature, and can be changed to start flowering as soon as you'd like."

Herban Legend had only a few in stock and they were very droopy, sad looking little things. But I bought them anyway and returned home to San Diego. My husband and I were worried about what would happen if we were pulled over because, although I had my medical marijuana card for California, the plants are still not legal according to federal law. But since this was the holy grail of cannabis plants, we decided to take the risk. Besides, it wouldn't be like driving across one of those zero-tolerance states. Californians had voted yes to proposition 215.

We made it back safely to San Diego with our little plants and took them over to a friend who happened to be a marijuana grower. He said they were weak genetically and in bad shape but thought he could revive them. Unfortunately, when he had to go out of town for a few days, a cold snap hit and the plants died.

Next I decided to grow some regular high-THC plants indoors. We set up a little enclosed area with a powerful grow light and the plants grew nice and strong. But I became nervous after a while when our electric bill spiked. I was afraid that would trigger law enforcement to search our home. I was probably being overly paranoid since I had my card and the right number of plants, according to CA state law. But in any case, fear got the best of me and I abandoned the project.

"I don't think the high-THC plants would have worked anyway. Dr. Courtney said it should be a high-CBD strain," I told my husband.

I decided to try several high-CBD oils and tinctures, but I never experienced any relief from them whatsoever.

When discussing the juicing leaf idea with another grower friend, he said, "I would be curious to see if it works. I'll bring you the trimmings I have so you can try it."

My husband was certain that it was worth juicing any leaf I could find but I didn't believe him. At that time, the only information we had was Dr. Courtney's recommendation to juice ACDC 22:1. He said I should plant a clone every day and juice one clone and one or two buds daily from the plant. It could take up to six months to see results, he added.

More research revealed that Kristen Courtney in the beginning juiced whatever leaf she could obtain. So I tried it. Our friend brought over a little bag of leaf. I thanked him politely but as I eyed the small bag, I doubted that it could yield much juice. Nevertheless, I put it through my wheatgrass juicer and it yielded enough juice to last for a couple of days. I drank it but didn't notice any improvements.

A few weeks later he brought over a huge garbage bag full of fresh leaf. It was beautiful, healthy looking leaf with a pungent aroma. I was eager to pull the leaves from the stems and juice it all as quickly as possible. I figured that once it was in juice form and frozen in my freezer, there was little risk because no one would know what it was. And the smell would be contained once it was juiced, poured into ice cube trays, and sealed within plastic bags in my freezer.

So I popped a few cubes into a glass each day and mixed it with freshly juiced apples and carrots. I didn't notice any change during the first three days. Then I started feeling more energy and experienced great elimination. And I didn't need any Advil for the next four days! My elimination was better than I had ever experienced. The funny thing is that after going to the bathroom, I left behind a very distinct aroma. It smelled exactly like someone lit up a joint.

Then, sadly, I ran out of leaf. My friend could not supply me with more because of a spider mite infestation in his crops. After that, the leaf delivery ceased.

"How can we do this so that we get all the leaf we need without any risk to us?" I asked my husband in frustration. In life I've found that it's very important to ask the right questions and frame them in a positive way, even and especially when you're frustrated. Because once you set your intention and ask a positive question, your mind goes to work finding the best possible answer to the question.

"Look on the Internet for hemp juice," he said.

"Hemp juice? No one is going to be juicing hemp," I said.

"Well, if they are, it should be legal to bring into the United States because we already import hemp fabric, hemp protein powders, hemp cereal, hemp oil—you just can't grow it here yet."

Few people understand the difference between hemp and cannabis. The short story is that hemp is cannabis but a different strain than marijuana. It is a more fibrous and leggy plant, used for many things such as paper, rope and cloth production. It is a great soil amendment and rotation crop as well. George Washington used to grow hemp when hemp could even be used to pay your taxes! It generally contains 1% to 1.5% CBDa and 0.1% to 0.3% THCa.

Anyway, it was worth a look. To my surprise there was a new company in the Netherlands that was offering flash frozen industrial hemp juice. But they were only offering it to European Union countries. I wrote to them anyway and they agreed to try to sell it to us here in the US with the stipulation that we had to take full responsibility if the shipment was held up and rejected by customs officials. And this stuff was not cheap, especially because of the $500 shipping bill. But the more I researched hemp juice, the more I became convinced that it could help me and others here in the US. It was worth the risk.

After about a month of making numerous phone calls and getting the paperwork we needed from the USDA and FDA, the package was shipped. But, as we had anticipated, it was delayed in customs. The FDA wanted to inspect its label. Since the frozen juice was on dry ice, time was of the essence. But there was absolutely nothing we could do to expedite the process.

Fortunately, the package was released after 24 hours and made it to our home five days after shipping. I drank 8 ounces of the juice per day for almost a month with minimal results. The juice was very thin, with a weak odor. I suspected that it might have been watered down. My elimination was a little better and I had slightly more energy but I was still experiencing significant pain. Ultimately, I felt like I wasted a good deal of money.

It's very challenging to persevere day in, day out without seeing major results, especially when that action hits your pocketbook hard. But I know from my research that it can take a while to see healing from the juice because it needs to saturate and accumulate in your fatty tissues.

In the meantime, I started taking hemp oil in capsules and CBD sublingual drops. I found no relief from them whatsoever. Next, I tried whole seed hemp protein powder. I figured that I should try to start saturating my body with cannabinoids, even minimally, until such time that I would have leaf to juice again. I actually did see some result from this very affordable powder (Vitacost Organic Hemp Protein High Fiber Drink Mix.)

The first time I took it I mixed it with some yogurt and honey and had it in the early evening. Then I had the worst insomnia ever. I couldn't figure it out. I hadn't had coffee that afternoon. So I searched on some forums on the Internet and found someone who was taking the same thing to help control epileptic seizures. He said that he never takes it in the evening because it gives him insomnia!

I later learned that whole seed hemp powder comes from industrial hemp seed, which is a sativa strain so it naturally gives you energy. So I began taking it first thing in the morning for breakfast and it did give me a boost in energy. Still had a lot of pain but my energy gain was somewhat noticeable.

Since my chronic pain was still significant, I resumed research on the Internet trying to find someone who would sell me the juice from an industrial hemp plant or even regular marijuana. I thought I'd give the hemp juice another go, thinking that perhaps since it's relatively low in CBDa that I just needed to drink it for a longer period of time. Maybe I hadn't given it a long enough trial period.

Eventually my search turned up a small family company in Ireland. They grew just a small amount of industrial hemp biodynamically, juiced it using a masticating juicer, flash froze it, and shipped the product throughout the UK. I contacted them and we set up a shipment to the US. This time, though, the package was held up for an entire month and subsequently destroyed. The main problem was the faulty packaging and labeling, which the company is now trying to rectify. The juice arrived half melted and leaking everywhere.

Even in its melted form, I did notice a huge difference between this juice and the one from the Netherlands. This one was very pungent smelling, almost as strong as the marijuana juice I had consumed before. And it was dark green and thick. I didn't drink any of it, though, for fear of contamination.

I felt profoundly despondent. What was I going to do now? Should I just give in to modern medicine and take some pill? Everything I had heard from people I know who have RA or people I read about with RA suggested that they all experienced adverse side effects from pharmaceuticals and/or the meds just stopped working after a while. This was not the route I wanted to go but I was in so much pain and misery, I had to do something.

My husband texted our grower friend again and explained the situation. "Do you have any leaf available for us?" he asked. This time the answer was yes! It was harvest time and there was a lot of leaf available. He brought me enough to last a few months with more expected in the coming months. I was extremely grateful.

It took me two days to process all the leaf through the juicer in part because of frequent clogging. I had to remove all the hard stems first before juicing. I poured all the juice into ice cube trays and started drinking it daily. Then the miracle happened. I started to heal!

By day 12 I was 80% better than I was before I started. Before I started I was taking anywhere from 1 to 4 Advil pills per day and 1 to 3 droppers of cannabis-infused olive oil (see Chapter 10, Cannabis Oil, Tincture & Salve). I would wake up about 10 times a night in pain, having to take Advil and cannabis oil just so that I could fall back to sleep. All my joints were in pain, making it difficult to even get out of bed at night and walk to the bathroom.

All day long I would endure various stages of misery, drinking ginger tea to help quell the inflammation in my body. Of course, life goes on regardless of chronic pain. I had to work and help my husband take care of our kids. There was no stepping off the treadmill of life just because I didn't feel well. Besides, if I did quit and give in to my pain, I was afraid I'd never move forward and recover.

Again, during the first few days of juicing I didn't notice much change except for improved elimination. But I did find that I was getting high from the juice this time. Such a different response frightened me somewhat because I wasn't sure how high I would get. It was an unexpected and unintended side effect that did not occur the last time I juiced my friend's leaf for a week. During a brief phone consultation with Dr. Courtney, he mentioned that they had a similar result from juicing and he suspected that the leaf must have touched one of the grow lights, thus activating the THC. I suspect that's what had happened with my batch of leaf, too.

But I got around the high, mostly, by sipping the juice throughout the day, just a few sips at a time. The juice should be consumed this way anyway, according to Kristen, keeping it in your system at all times. Maybe it was just the plant's way of teaching me how to use it.

I continued to get mildly high during the day, which I really didn't like, but I pressed on because I was confident that the juice would help me. After a while, the juice made me a little high just on an occasional basis. I have no idea why the variation occurred from day to day. What I've noticed, for me, is that the longer I juice, the cleaner my diet needs to be and the more I need to manage my stress. Because if I eat junk or get stressed out, I really notice it. So the juice is amazing but you still have to live well to feel well.

By day 3 I didn't need any Advil. Each day I received a new little gift. Each night my sleep improved and each day my energy increased incrementally. On the morning of day 8, my 7-year-old daughter asked me to braid her hair. I didn't even think about it, I just braided her hair, and it looked great. Then I remembered that just a few months earlier when she had asked me to braid her hair, I couldn't even begin to do it. I cried then, feeling like a failure for having let her down and being unable to perform such an easy task. It sounds like such a little thing but I was buoyed all day by having been able to braid my daughter's hair this time around!

Every day is a little easier for me. I can move better in the mornings than I used to and sleep more soundly at night. Recently, I noticed that I climbed my stairs in the evening without pain or trouble. I was even able to perch on the balls of my feet. I'm able to use my fork properly again, even though I still have some swelling in my right wrist. I can cut vegetables on a cutting board without pain. And I no longer wake up drenched in sweat after taking Advil in the middle of the night as if a low-grade fever had broken. But this time around I have noticed that my stools are usually loose. I worried about this until we bought a dairy cow. The previous owner said that whenever the cow just eats grass in the field, she has diarrhea. When she eats hay, her stools are much more firm. So perhaps the looseness in my stool is due to drinking "grass"!

On a recent beautiful spring evening I had the urge to go for a run. I hadn't felt like doing that in years. So I did! Well, sort of. My feet still hurt and my right knee is swollen but I took my younger daughter with me and we did a shuffle down the street. Then we came home and did 20 minutes of yoga and meditated. Afterwards she said to me, "This was the best day ever!" I need no more motivation than that to continue drinking this juice so I can completely heal.

The beneficial healing effects of CBDa and cannabinoids are thought to be derived from extended saturation in the body. But I've noticed that when I delay drinking the juice until later in the day, I feel slight pain. When I drink the juice, the pain subsides. So the juice does seem to exert a short-term pain-relieving effect as well as a long-term healing effect.

By day 55, I'd estimate that I've improved by about 85%. Of course, this is subjective and unscientific, but I can safely say that while I'm still stiff and somewhat sore in the early mornings, my discomfort fades away much quicker. And then there's joint damage that needs to be repaired and that should take more time. But since I began juicing I no longer get the "icky" inflamed feeling I used to feel intermittently all day. Unless I eat too much sugar or pork.

I think the reason I haven't fully healed yet is because I'm taking a very low dose (1 to 3 ounces daily) of the juice so that I don't get high and to conserve my supply. I listen to my body and take what feels right. If I had grown the leaf myself and knew that it would not get me high, I would be drinking 8 ounces daily and probably already be fully healed. But I am still extremely grateful for my progress and I feel certain that I will get to full remission in the near future.

So why am I writing this book when I haven't completely healed? Well, most people with chronic pain that I know would give their right arm to have the results I've achieved with this juice in such a short time period without adverse side effects. How many people who pop pills can boast of similar results? And I am not taking any pharmaceuticals or cannabis oil at all.

Now you may be wondering if drinking this juice until you heal is sufficient or whether continuing indefinitely is necessary. The answer is you have to keep going. According to the Courtneys, when the juicing ceases, the disease symptoms can return. I don't know if that's true for everyone but when I met with Dr. Courtney in person he said I'd have to juice for life. And based on my short one-week trial months ago, I think that demonstrated relapse occurs without the juice. I felt better on day 4, needing no more pain medication, and then by day 8 when I ran out of juice, I slipped back into needing medication again.

Living with and trying to treat my RA has felt like a long, arduous journey. I am by no means an expert on dietary cannabis but I am a believer in its use as a patient and consumer. Other than Kristen's YouTube video there is little information available on its dietary/medical use on the Internet, especially testimonials. I'm not sure why but I speculate that perhaps either a) people are not juicing it due to the difficulty in obtaining the juice (or the whole plant/leaves) or b) some normally law-abiding yet sick citizens are consuming it and seeing results but they don't wish to publicize it for fear of being punished by law enforcement.

I mulled these ideas and the risks involved before choosing to share this with you. I think in life sometimes you have to stand up for what you believe in, stand up for what is right. I wrote this book to help fill in the gaps of information on this topic in easy-to-understand language. And to give hope, in the form of a personal testimonial, to the millions of people in the world who are sick and can be helped by this amazing plant. Testimonials can be very psychologically powerful in the healing process. As I obtain more testimonials (perhaps from you!) I will include them in this book. So please write me at katie@juicingcannabisforhealing.com.

The Courtneys are bravely leading the way and shedding light on the healing capabilities of cannabis. But they are just two people. Two people can only do and share so much. Especially two people who are parents to several small children! Maybe you are like me in that you saw their video, became interested in learning more about dietary cannabis but couldn't find any more information on the topic that wasn't just a regurgitation of the Courtney's interview or a dense scientific paper. I hope to bridge that gap and give you all the information I have found through trial and error as well as keep you up to date on any new information that comes along. If you would like to be emailed a free updated PDF copy of this book, just send me an email, katie@juicingcannabisforhealing.com.

I believe this plant has been put on our beautiful planet for us, and other creatures, to consume in order to attain optimal health. They say if you want to be healthy and heal, look no further than your front yard. There are many edible plants in our yards that most of us don't even know about. This knowledge has been lost, for the most part, over the generations. We think we need to go to the grocery store to eat. We don't. My family and I live on a burgeoning sustainable farm that is off grid. We are learning how to live off the land and from our animals. It's an interesting process with a steep learning curve but I think what we are learning is extremely valuable. Not just for the future of our small family but for the future of our planet.

We've been so conditioned to give our power away to medical professionals and pharmaceutical companies. When you get sick, what is the first thing you do? Pop a pill? Ride it out? Look within and try to figure out the cause? The other day my younger daughter asked me, "Mommy, why did you get sick? How did you get arthritis?" I told her that I didn't know. But I started thinking more about it. I think I do know. It was stress. Stress was the trigger anyway. Perhaps there was a low-lying infection that my body could fight and handle until I put myself under too much stress. Then my body couldn't handle it and a disease process started.

What if instead of turning to the doctor immediately we turned to our own inner wisdom? And combine that with stress-relieving exercises, such as yoga and meditation, coupled with natural herbs and healthful whole foods and you may have yourself a prescription for healing. You can grow your own medicine. You have the power, and now the tools, to heal yourself.

Chapter 5
Some of the Diseases Cannabis Juice Helps Alleviate and/or Put into a Sustained Remission

Juicing with cannabis can lead to "sustained remission" but usually not a "cure" in the sense that you need to continue consuming the juice to achieve remission and remain in a state of good health. But as long as you continue to drink it, once you achieve sustained remission, I suspect it will certainly feel like a cure. But every individual is different so it's not completely out of the realm of possibility that you will achieve a full cure from the juice and not have to continue juicing. Most people do have to continue juicing to stay healthy.

Some of the diseases I list below have been shown in various medical studies to respond favorably to medical marijuana via smoking, vaporizing, and/or consuming baked goods containing marijuana ("edibles"); most are only anecdotally known to help alleviate disease symptoms. But, in my opinion, anecdotal evidence is nothing to ignore. After all, my story is anecdotal. It's real people finding incredible relief through unconventional means.

Please keep in mind that this is not a list of diseases that are known to resolve from juicing cannabis. There is not much of that going on at the moment due to lack of education, availability of leaf, and scientific studies. But I think it stands to reason that if people with these conditions are reporting relief from decarboxylated cannabis, they would experience considerable relief if many of the beneficial cannabinoids and terpenes were not destroyed! Terpenes are what give cannabis its distinct aroma. Like cannabinoids, they have considerable and unique healing properties of their own.

Imagine if people suffering from these diseases not only received temporary relief but were able to actually put their disease *into long-term sustained remission?* This is possible, with some diseases, by juicing cannabis. How many of these diseases, at this time, is unknown.

This list has been culled from an excellent website: http://medicalmarijuana.com/treatments-with-medical-marijuana-cannabis. If you go to the website and click on the disease you are interested in learning more about, you will be directed to a page that gives you detailed information about the disease's symptoms, which strains work best for it, and a list of supportive papers, articles, or studies, if any, that are available.

So, finally, here is the list:

Acute Gastritis

Addiction

Adenomyosis

Alzheimer's Disease

Amyloidosis

Amyotrophic Lateral Sclerosis (ALS) [also known as Lou Gehrig's disease]

Anaphylactic Shock or Reaction

Angelman Syndrome

Anorexia

Arthritis

Arthropathy (Gout)

Asperger Disorder

Asthma

Attention Deficit Disorder (ADD)

Autism

Back Pain

Bell's Palsy

Bipolar Disorder

Bruxism

Bulimia

Cachexia

Cancer

Carpal Tunnel Syndrome

Cerebral Aneurysm

Chronic Fatigue Syndrome (CFS)

Chronic Pain

Cluster Headaches

Charcot-Marie-Tooth (CMT) Disease

Colitis/Ulcerative Colitis

Colon Diverticulitis

Crohn's disease

Cyclic Vomiting Syndrome (CVS)

Cystic Fibrosis

Cystitis/Urethritis

Darier's Disease

Depression

Diabetes

Diarrhea

Dravet Syndrome

Dupuytren's Contracture

Dyspepsia

Dystonia

Essential Thrombocythemia (ET)

Eczema

Ehlers-Danlos Syndrome

Emphysema

Endometriosis

Epilepsy/Seizure Disorder

Felty's Syndrome

Fibromyalgia

Friedreich's Ataxia

Gastroesophageal Reflux Disease

Glaucoma

Graves' Disease

Hemophilia A

Henoch-Schonlein Purpura

Herpes

HIV/AIDS
Hydrocephalus
Hypertension (High Blood Pressure)
Hyperventilation
Hypoglycemia
Incontinence
Inflammatory Bowel Disease
Insomnia
Interstitial Pneumonia
Irritable Bowel Syndrome
Limbic Rage Syndrome
Liver Disease
Lupus
Lyme Disease
Macular Degeneration
Marfan Syndrome
Mastocytosis
Melorheostosis
Meniere's Disease
Menopausal Syndrome
Methamphetamine Syndrome
Methicillian-Resistant Staphylococcus Aureus (MRSA)
Migraines
Motion Sickness
Movement Disorders
Multiple Sclerosis (MS)
Muscular Dystrophy (MD)
Muscle Spasm

Myofascial Pain

Nausea

Nephritis

Neurodegenerative Disorders

Neurofibromatosis

Neuropathy

Nightmares

Nail Patella Syndrome

Osgood-Schlatter Syndrome

Osteogenesis Imperfecta

Palmar Hyperhydrosis

Pancreatic Cancer

Pancreatitis

Panic Attacks

Panic Disorder

Patellofemoral Pain Syndrome

Pectus Carinatum (Pigeon breast/chest)

Pemphigus

Peptic Ulcer

Peutz-Jehgers Syndrome

Polyarteritis Nodosa

Polycythemia Vera

Porphyria—Alternative Symptom Treatments

Post-Concussion Syndrome

Post-Traumatic Stress Disorder (PTSD)

PPS-Post Polio Syndrome (PPS)

Prostate Cancer

Pruritus

Psoriasis

Pylorospasm Reflux

Radiation Therapy

Raynaud's Phenomenon

Reactive Arthritis

Restless Leg Syndrome

Social Anxiety Disorder (SAD)

Schizophrenia(s)

Scleroderma

Scoliosis

Selectivemutism

Shingles

Sinusitis

Sjogren's Syndrome

Sleep Apnea

Spina Bifida

Sturge-Weber Syndrome

Syringomyelia

Tenosynovitis

Testicular Cancer

Testicular Torsion

Thoracic Outlet Syndrome

Tietze's Syndrome

Tinnitus

Tourette Syndrome

Trigeminal Neuralgia (TN), also known as Tic Douloureux

Trichotillomania (also known as Trichotillosis or Hair Pulling Disorder)

This list is almost laughably extensive. Is there really such thing as a panacea? What on earth could possibly help with so many different diseases? Well, I'm here to tell you that I'm not laughing. I feel like dropping to my knees every day in tears of overwhelming gratitude for how much better it makes me feel. It is truly the tree, or plant, of life.

Unfortunately, we live in a corrupt world where governments and pharmaceutical companies are bedfellows. Consider all the jobs that are created within certain government law enforcement institutions that exist solely to fight the use of cannabis. Think about the benefits that alcohol purveyors derive from keeping cannabis marginalized. Alcohol, after all, is considered by scientists to be much more detrimental than cannabis, with far fewer known benefits.

Pharmaceutical companies cannot make money from selling raw plant juice. So they pick out the most beneficial molecule, make an artificial copy of it, put it into a pill and sell it to us. But it doesn't work. Just ask anyone who has tried Marinol (the artificial pharmaceutical version of THC).

In the next chapter I will attempt to explain some of the science behind the cannabinoids, as I understand it, in layperson's terms.

Chapter 6
How Cannabinoids Work

In December 2004, *Scientific American* published an article titled "The Brain's Own Marijuana." This was the inspiration for Dr. Courtney's discovery of dietary cannabis. Medical schools historically have taught students that neurotransmitters offer one-way traffic. This means that they can fire off signals but not receive information. So when the immune system becomes imbalanced, like it does in autoimmune disorders, the body erroneously attacks its own healthy tissues.

But this is not necessarily true. The endocannabinoid system within the human brain produces cannabinoids like those found in cannabis and breast milk. These cannabinoids send information back to the neurotransmitters, giving them information about what's going on in the body and allowing for a self-modulating feedback loop.

However, when a disease process develops, this feedback loop is altered or severed. It can be replaced externally through the introduction into the body of cannabinoids such as those found in mother's milk or cannabis. CB1 receptors are all over the body, especially in the brain. The body makes its own cannabinoids called endocannabinoids but in small quantities that rapidly degrade.

There is much ongoing discovery related to endocannabinoids. (http://bit.ly/WkHTYb)

A relatively new theory, posited by Dr. Ethan Russo of GW Pharmaceuticals in the UK, suggests that some people become ill with the diseases mentioned in the previous chapter simply because they have a clinical endocannabinoid deficiency (CECD). In other words, their brains don't create sufficient levels of health regulating cannabinoids they need to stay healthy.
(http://wapo.st/1po7uHL)

I find it very interesting that cannabis contains over 421 chemical compounds, including **80 phytocannabinoids that have not been found in any other plant.**
(http://www.cannabisinternational.org/info/Non-Psychoactive-Cannabinoids.pdf)

It is also notable that the greatest source of endogenous cannabinoids, meaning those that your body produces, is found in mother's breast milk.
(http://bit.ly/WkHTYb)

There is a chart at http://www.cannabisinternational.org/about.php that can help you to get an understanding of what cannabinoids can do for you. These are the non-heated cannabinoids.

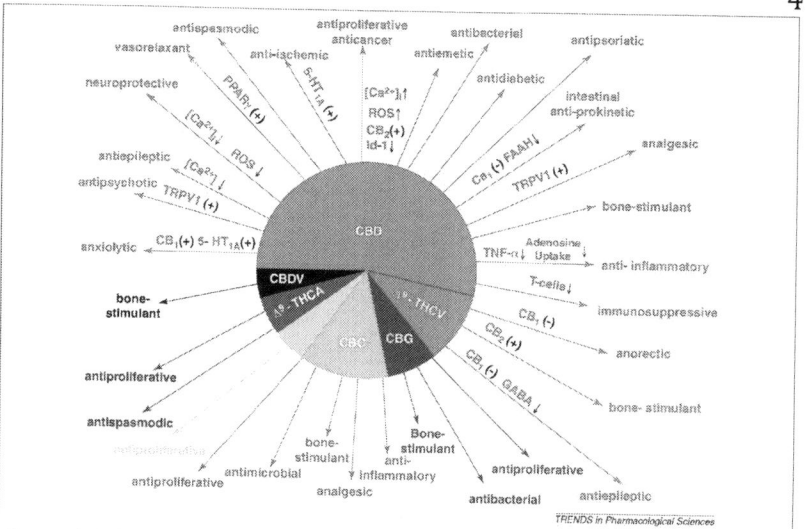

Pharmacological actions of non-psychotropic cannabinoids (with the indication of the proposed mechanisms of action)
Abbreviations: D9-THC, D9-tetrahydrocannabinol; D8-THC, D8-tetrahydrocannabinol; CBN, cannabinol; CBD, cannabidiol; D9-THCV, D9-tetrahydrocannabivarin; CBC, cannabichromene; CBG, cannabigerol; D9-THCA, D9-tetrahydrocannabinolic acid; CBDA, cannabidiolic acid; TRPV1, transient receptor potential vanilloid type 1; PPARg, peroxisome proliferator-activated receptor g; ROS, reactive oxygen species; 5-HT1A, 5-hydroxytryptamine receptor subtype 1A; FAAH, fatty acid amide hydrolase. (+), direct or indirect activation; ↑, increase; ↓, decrease.

The Journal of Cannabis in Clinical Practice by O'Shaughnessy can be found in some health food stores or online. This journal is a great resource for learning which cannabis strains are good for particular conditions and what percent of the various cannabinoids they contain. (http://www.beyondthc.com/print-edition/)

As I mentioned in Chapter 2, Why Juice It?, in order for the THCa and CBDa to be converted to THC and CBD, the plant must be dried over a long period of time or, to speed up the process, you heat the plant. This heating and drying process is known as decarboxylation. According to marijuanagrowershq.com (http://bit.ly/1sAD9em), "Decarboxylation is a chemical reaction that releases carbon dioxide (CO_2). This means a chemical reaction takes place in which carboxylic acids loose [sic] a carbon atom from a carbon chain. This process converts THCA to THC, the much loved compound with many medicinal and psychoactive effects. When the cannabis dries, it very, very slowly begins to decarboxylate and converts THCA to THC.

"The good news is we don't have to wait years for cannabis to decarboxylate. We can speed things along with a process that is a lot simpler than you might expect. Simply heating dried cannabis to the correct temperature for enough time releases that carbon dioxide and creates THC."

So as you can see, decarboxylation is a result of heat over time, or just drying the plant out over time. For our purposes, we just need to have a basic understanding of decarboxylation and why to avoid it. The temperature and the amount of time required to decarboxylate each cannabinoid or terpene varies significantly. My research revealed that the lowest temperature where decarboxylation takes place is 212 F.

I was recently asked if you can put the cannabis leaves into a dehydrator and make "cannabis chips." Given that decarboxylation is a function of time and temperature, basically drying out the plant, I would say no. But because it appears that 212 F is the lowest temperature at which decarboxylation takes place, and most dehydrators heat fruits, vegetables, and meats between 130 F and 155 F, it may be possible if you consume it right away. But I don't know for certain. If you wait a while before eating the dehydrated leaves, it seems to me that the leaves would continue to decarboxylate over time. To be safe (i.e., not get too high), I wouldn't try it. But if you try it, do so carefully and please let me know your results so I can inform others. In any case, cannabis chips would be an acquired taste, likely, even if you seasoned it with a bunch of sea salt!

Israeli cannabinoid researchers Shimon Ben-Shabat and Raphael Mechoulam came up with a theory called The Entourage Effect. Basically it states that all chemical compounds within the cannabis plant work best together. Therefore, CBD works better with THC present. When you try to extract one compound, such as CBD, it won't be as effective as it is when in perfect balanced synergy within the whole plant.

I contacted Dr. Raphael Mechoulam via email to try to get more answers about acidic cannabinoids. He indicated that the acidic cannabinoids, such as THCa and CBDa, are very unstable and easily convert to THC and CBD. This may happen if the juice has been sitting around for some time. But he added, "Please note that there is very little research published on the cannabinoid acids, although we identified them about 50 years ago. We know that they do not cause psychoactivity. Most research published is on CBD and THC; almost nothing on the acids."

I'm inclined to think that he's right about the juice sitting around and converting from THCa to THC. The only batch of leaf that I've ever gotten high from happened after I left it in the fridge for too many days. In fact, some of it turned rather rancid tasting. It's difficult to say how many days it would take to possibly flip over to THC, but I think the safest thing to do is to either a) consume the juice right away or b) freeze it. I've had no problems with any juice that I have frozen immediately.

If you would like to delve deeper and learn more about what research has been done with cannabis, please check out this website of Clinical Studies and Case Reports (http://tinyurl.com/lytwr66). On this website you will find "clinical studies with cannabis or single cannabinoids in different diseases and case reports on the use of cannabis by patients. You may search for diseases (indications), authors, medication, study design (controlled study, open trial, case report, etc.) and other criteria."

Chapter 7
Suggested Dosage

How much cannabis is enough? There have been no studies performed on people, to my knowledge, using raw cannabis juice. All the government studies and patents have been based on isolating the CBD or THC molecules. Researchers have not studied the synergistic effects of all of the known cannabinoids and terpenes together in the raw plant.

There was an informal juice study conducted with about 12 patients at the Humboldt Patient Resource Center in Northern California. Investigators gave patients free cannabis leaf and wheatgrass juicers. Most of the patients had arthritis. Patients were assisted in changing their diets to become more alkaline and were guided to incorporate yoga into their lives as well. After 90 days of juicing just 1 ounce per day of whatever fresh, raw leaf they could obtain, all patients improved tremendously. Some of the patients even observed noticeable gains before 90 days.

According to laboratory research, the rule of thumb for dosing is 1 to 40 mg of CBDa per 1 kilogram (kg) of body weight per day. (http://www.cannabisinternational.org/info/treatingyourself.pdf)

So since I'm 120 pounds, or almost 55 kg, I would need to consume anywhere from 55 mg to 2,200 mg of CBDa daily. But this guideline is based on isolating the synthetic version of the CBDa molecule in a lab. I suspect that much less is needed when the CBDa is balanced with all of the other cannabinoids and terpenes in the raw leaf. Besides, how does one know how much CBDa is in one ounce of juice? Well, it depends on how you obtain it. If you grow it yourself and juice it, you would have to find a cannabis lab to test the contents and then figure out the math from there.

I recommend just trying it to see how it works for you. If you can only obtain 1 ounce of juice per day of unknown CBD concentration, don't worry. Just know that it may take longer for the cannabis to saturate your fatty tissues and exert its healing magic. Six to eight ounces of raw cannabis juice per day is a good rule of thumb for sick people. Dr. Courtney believes that everyone should drink cannabis juice throughout their entire lives because preventing illness is so much easier than curing it.

There's another very informal rule of thumb that I've found to help me gauge my dosage. If my poop smells like pot, then I figure my body is fully saturated. If it doesn't smell like pot, then I probably need to up my dosage. It can take a day or two of increased juice consumption before you notice a change in smell.

Also sometimes you may be going along in your life feeling great when changes in your environment, such as a big winter storm or stress can bring on a flare up. I have had a few flare ups since juicing but they have been much easier to handle than before. And only one was kind of memorable. To get through these times you can do three things: one, increase your juice consumption; two, do very gentle exercise such as tai chi and qi gong; and, three, consider changing strains. Whether it's a strain high in CBD or high in THC, whatever you can get hold of, just give it a try. You can always go back to your original strain after the flare up passes. Changing strains may not work for everyone but it is worth a try and it should cause you no harm as long as it's leaf that hasn't been sprayed by chemicals.

I once asked Dr. Courtney if hemp juice would work like marijuana leaf. He said yes. He had heard from a young patient who had wonderful results. But as I said, in my experience, it did not work (though I am not sure of the quality of the supply I purchased). I also spoke with someone in California who had juiced hemp. He has ankylosing spondylitis and had wonderful results with hemp juice. Then he had to move and was unable to grow more hemp, leading to the resumption of his pain.

The biggest question in my mind is what role THCa plays in the synergistic relationship between the various cannabinoids. In other words, was the CBDa too low in the hemp or was the THCa too low? Or was it one of the other reasons I have mentioned before?

All of the research has been done in the lab on synthetic cannabinoids, not on the plant itself because of current federal law.

The one exception is an oral spray pharmaceutical called Sativex. This product is used to help alleviate the spasticity associated with multiple sclerosis. It is available in Canada, the UK, and New Zealand but not in the US because it contains the real cannabinoids THC and CBD.

One thing to keep in mind is that anyone can have an allergy to anything. Even cannabis. So when you begin, start with a very small dose. If you tolerate it well, inch it up from there. Interestingly, hemp has been shown to repair damaged DNA due to two proteins: edestin and albumin. It is believed that edestin is only found in hemp seeds and it is very similar to blood plasma. You can receive the benefits from these DNA-repairing proteins by even just consuming raw hemp seeds or hemp seed oil. (http://www.hightimes.com/read/hemp-repairs-damaged-dna)

I had a few lingering questions that I could not resolve from my research. Trying to get hold of the Courtneys is very difficult and there are very few dietary cannabis experts in the world. One is Dr. Ethan Russo. I emailed him but did not receive a response. So I reached out to Igor Grant, MD, who works at the UC San Diego Center for Medicinal Cannabis Research (CMCR). He was unavailable for questions but the co-director of CMCR, J. H. Atkinson, MD, agreed to answer some of my questions. The only two questions Dr. Atkinson had answers to are listed below for your information.

KM: If someone consumes the raw cannabis plant in the form of juice (and presuming it has not been heated so it only contains THCa), would that person be able to pass a drug test for THC?

Dr. Atkinson: The person will test positive for cannabinoids (urine, blood).

KM: How do ratios work? For instance, there's a plant, ACDC 22:1 that has 22 parts CBDa to 1 part THCa. If an industrial hemp plant contains 1.5% CBDa and 0.3% THCa, then what would be the ratio of CBDa to THCa? (Sorry, I know this is more of a math question but it's beyond my abilities at the moment.)

Dr. Atkinson: If I understand your question, the ratio you describe is 5:1.

KM: If the effective dose of CBDa is 1 to 40 milligrams to 1 kilogram of body weight, how can this be measured on a practical level when one is juicing a plant?

Dr. Atkinson: I don't know how precise one can be at the crude level of juicing. Also, since there is very wide variation among people in rates of absorption and elimination of cannabinoids delivered to the gut (ingested), with there being an 8-fold variation, for example, in time to onset of action (e.g., 1 hour for some people, 8 hours for others) a given 'dose' may perform differently depending on the individual (e.g., duration of action varies likewise).

When growing your own plants or when you obtain leaf from others, try to get leaf that is from the vegetative state versus the flowering state. The reason for this is that it is more potent in vegetative state. As the plant begins the budding process, it draws energy and nutrients from the leaf and puts it into the bud. I believe that's why many of the leaves turn yellow as the buds grow.

When you are growing your own, you can do this by extracting leaf and branches from the bottom of the plant first as that is the area that gets the least amount of sunlight and therefore only offers popcorn-sized buds anyway. As the buds begin to develop, remove as much leaf as you can without causing the plant to go into shock. Remember that the plant does need some leaf because the leaves are its solar collectors. I would do this process over the course of days and monitor your plants to see how they tolerate the leaf removal.

You can even juice male plants as the pollen sacks are beneficial and the male plants are thought to be as potent as the females with regard to juicing or eating the plant. Sometimes growers will discover male plants and wish to destroy them. If you network with some growers, you could be the beneficiary of these male plants. You're helping the grower out and they're definitely helping you!

Chapter 8
Where to Get the Juice

One day perhaps we'll be able to go to our local health food store and buy hemp or cannabis juice by the gallon in the refrigerated or frozen food sections in packets. But today it's not so easy. You can obtain it but you will probably have to be patient and persistent. I am going to present you with the various options. I'm not advocating that you take any particular actions; I'm just telling you what's available.

Contact a Juice Supplier

This option is only good if you live in or can move to Oregon or Colorado, as these companies cannot ship out of state. I am sure there will be more companies offering this soon, but for now this is all the information I have. I have not tried their juice as I do not reside in either of these states. So I can't vouch for them. If you hear of any other companies offering this, please let me know so I can share it with everyone.

CannaSqueezed
Jamie
Denver, Colorado
720-982-0272
720-757-4413

cannasqueezed@gmail.com

(You can also look them up on FaceBook)

Cannabis Angels
Dan
Portland, Oregon
971-221-9391
cannabisangels.com
cannabisangels@gmail.com

Contact a Local Grower

This option is good if you don't have any seeds or clones at your immediate disposal, and if you don't have any personal experience growing marijuana. A local grower could be a medical marijuana dispensary servicing your area, a local caregiver, or even your cousin's friend's brother who has a grow room for his and his friends' personal use. Some growers advertise on craigslist to sell their clones.

I recently learned that growers pick the fan leaves from the cannabis plant a few days before they harvest the bud. This temporarily shocks the plant and then it pours all of its energy into expanding the bud for survival. Most growers don't even compost the leaf; they just *throw it away* primarily because of the odor. Some do make hash out of the leaf but most of the time they just toss it away. A grower needs to be as discreet as possible and that means controlling indoor growing aromas. This is usually accomplished with an ozone or carbon filter but anything that can be done to weaken the smell is a good idea.

It is worth noting that the cannabis plant is much less fragrant during the vegetative, or leafy, phase and much more pungent during the flowering, or budding, phase. In any case, since most growers just dispose of the leaf, you may find a grower that will give it to you for free or for a reasonable negotiated price. It can't hurt to ask.

The only problem with this option is that you are dependent on other people. And other people, as well meaning as they may be, can let you down. Or their crops can let you down. Sometimes plant diseases or spider mites or similar factors may interfere to render the leaf ineffective for juicing. If you grow your own, you'll have more control over these potential obstacles. Some dispensaries (in California, for instance) will actually sell you clones of the plant. Consider yourself lucky in such a situation. Just read about how to make it grow and you're good to go.

Buy Hemp Juice from a Supplier
To date and to my knowledge there are only two suppliers in the world offering frozen hemp juice. I've purchased from both of them and imported the frozen hemp juice into the US. As I mentioned earlier, the first supplier was from the Netherlands and their juice was extremely expensive and it did not help me at all. I drank it for a month. It was packaged well, but the juice was watery and had a weak, barely detectable aroma. This is not to say it won't

help you but I personally would not recommend this company as I also had the sense that their business practices amounted to price gouging.

The second company, as I also noted earlier, was a small hemp farm located in Ireland. Their product was much less expensive than the Dutch juice but the cost to ship it was still very expensive (more than $500 USD for a two-month supply just for the shipping). At the time this book went to press, they were growing their second batch of hemp and planned to harvest and juice it toward the end of summer. They use a masticating juicer for maximum extraction. And they are working on improving their packaging and streamlining the shipping process. But I don't think they'll be ready to deliver juice to anyone in the US just yet.

Call a University

When this book was printed, there were 23 US states plus the District of Columbia that allow people who are sick to have access to medical marijuana. The laws vary greatly from state to state and at this time federal law prohibits use and cultivation of marijuana. When state and federal laws clash, it creates a bit of a mess.

If your state allows you to have a medical marijuana card and grow some cannabis for your own personal use, and you do so according to their rules, will the federal government leave you alone? They are supposed to. As of mid December 2014, the huge 1.1 trillion dollar spending bill in the US effectively ended the prohibition in states that allow for medical marijuana by no longer giving funding to the

Drug Enforcement Agency (DEA) and other agencies to seek out and prosecute patients, caregivers, and dispensaries who are following their state's rules. You can read an article about it here: http://www.hightimes.com/read/congress-effectively-ends-federal-ban-medical-marijuana.

In the eyes of the federal government, is there a difference between growing regular marijuana and growing hemp? No, not at this time. However, the 2014 Farm Bill allows for certain state departments of agriculture to work in conjunction with state universities to grow industrial hemp for research purposes. Some universities are just getting started in growing their first hemp crops. Please see Appendix C, US States Allowed to Grow Hemp for Research as Per the 2014 US Farm Bill.

If you live in one of these states, you could call your state department of agriculture and ask if you can participate in their research studies on hemp. Explain that you wish to juice the leaf for health purposes. Show them a copy of this book, if you wish, and/or have them watch Kristen's video. I don't know if anyone has done this yet, but it's worth a try. If you do succeed, please send me an email (katie@juicingcannabisforhealing.com) so I can share this information with others.

Grow Your Own

I wonder why "weed" is one of the slang terms for cannabis. Does it grow easily like a weed? In my opinion, the term degrades the spirit of this incredible plant. But anyway, you can grow it indoors, outdoors in a greenhouse, or scatter plant it on your property or in the wild. "The wild" is probably not a great idea as it's more than frowned upon to grow it on land that is not yours. And bunnies will probably come eat it anyway if you don't protect it somehow in a structure.

How to grow cannabis is beyond the scope of this book. I have been growing my own high CBD cannabis to juice and I've made lots of mistakes. But they're still alive and budding and they are huge! So I know I'm doing something right. I've read lots of grow books, watched many YouTube grow videos, and read tons articles and forums. It's kind of difficult piecing together all the information and applying it to our specific dietary purposes. Our goals are different from most growers in that we want huge plants with lots of leaf as well as bud. Not just big buds.

I'm putting together an instructional grow package which will hopefully be available sometime in 2016. It will include a Grow Your Own Medicine to Juice video, Grow Your Own Medicine to Juice Instruction Manual, a list of doctors and licensed growers in the legal US mmj states, 21 Best Tasting Cannabis Smoothie Recipes, a paperback copy of this book, and free video updates for life.

I don't know about you, but for me I find it easier to learn when someone can just "show me" how to do something. There's a lot of cannabis grow videos on YouTube, but they're never the full deal. They only show bits and pieces about how to grow or about the various problems you may encounter when growing. And the vast majority of them do not speak to the medical home grower. I'm not an expert grower yet, but I have learned tons and I've been successful so far in growing my own medicine on a budget. I want to share with you what I've learned about how to easily and affordably grow cannabis indoors. If you want to be notified when this package is ready, shoot me an email at katie@juicingcannabisforhealing.com

Obviously it's faster to start growing from cuttings (clones) rather than seed and probably easier to obtain cuttings from a friend than it is to get seeds. Seeds are available for sale online from seed banks around the world (not in the US). Check out Appendix B, List of Seed Banks. But keep in mind that it's illegal to send and receive cannabis seeds through the mail in the US at this time. Seed companies do it anyway, with most using stealth packaging with guaranteed delivery. But it is a risk. If you do decide to purchase from a seed bank, consider the paper trail you leave if you pay via credit card. Many seed banks accept cash through the mail.

The US is rather schizophrenic regarding its stance on hemp; importation of hemp products is legal but growing it here, for now, remains illegal. A notable exception, as part of the Farm Bill, is cultivation at a university for research purposes. And even then, many states have been blocked from importing the seeds that they would need to begin their research.

You could try contacting Ryan Loflin in Colorado (www.facebook.com/ryan.loflin) and ask him if you could buy some leaf from him to juice. He's growing hundreds of acres of industrial hemp and he has a state permit to do so. Part of his crop will be made available for sale to the general public but before it leaves the state of Colorado it has to be processed in some form. I'd imagine frozen juice constitutes "processing," but I don't know for certain. He doesn't seem very enthusiastic about juicing, though. During a Twitter gathering I asked him if he would juice and ship it but I didn't get a response.

Start a Caregiver Chain

This idea is one way to spread the juice to all who need it. A "caregiver" in this instance is someone licensed with their state as a grower of cannabis. Every state has its own rules, but some states want the grower to provide medical marijuana card-carrying patients with buds, edibles, and topicals for a price. Each caregiver is usually limited to the number of patients they can grow for and the number of plants they can grow for each patient. In some states, it is legal to "gift" cuttings to another caregiver. In other words, money cannot change hands. In any case, if you become a caregiver, you can grow your own medicine and juice it and provide the juice to other patients. What we can do as caregivers is offer classes to our patients, showing them how to grow their own. And when they're ready, give them cuttings to start their garden.

Why would anyone start a business only to teach their customers how to become self-sufficient growers themselves? So that we can spread the knowledge and help others receive the juice. There will always be enough customers for the juice as long as you can educate people to its benefits. Also, cannabis doctors will refer patients to you, if their state law allows.

Chapter 9
Juicing Tips

At first glance, you may assume that you just need to plop the leaves into any juicer and out will come green juice. But remember that we do not want to heat up the cannabis and we need to extract the maximum amount of nutrients from this green gold. I used to use a masticating type juicer versus a centrifugal one. Centrifugal juicers have fast spinning metal blades that separate the juice from the pulp. They're the ones you see most often in stores and online. Centrifugal juicers could heat the juice and activate the THC while at the same time destroying some of the plant's beneficial enzymes, and get very clogged up in the juicing process.

Masticating juicers are slower than centrifugal juicers. The slow-turning screw crushes the plant material, thus releasing the juice without heating it up. If you just wish to extract the juice separate from the pulp, this is the way to go.

But now I have switched over to a Ninja. A Ninja is a very powerful blender that pulverizes and liquefies the cannabis, allowing you to consume the pulp along with the juice. It is like a Vitamix but a lot more affordable. If you choose to consume your cannabis in liquid form, this is the very best way to go because you won't be losing any of the cannabinoids, terpenes, and other beneficial molecules to the pulp that usually gets composted or tossed away.

When using a blender like a Ninja, you need to add a little water to make it blend well. You can put both leaf and bud in the Ninja with the water. When you go to pour it out, it's a bit chunky but you can still freeze the mixture in ice cube trays. And when it's time to make it into a smoothie, it blends up well the second time so that you almost don't notice the pulp.

Speaking of terpenes, according to growweedeasy.com, if you are growing your own medicine, there are several things you can do to increase terpene and terpenoid content in your cannabis. One of the things you can do is grow it in soil, not hydroponically. Although hydroponics may yield more buds, high quality composted soil will give you more powerful and greater terpene and terpenoid content. You can read their article about the many ways to increase terpene content here: http://www.growweedeasy.com/better-taste-better-smell.

If you don't have the money for a masticating juicer or a Vitamix, or you just happen to have some leaf to try but haven't had a chance to purchase one of these machines yet, you can put the leaf into a regular kitchen blender. Just add water, leaf, and blend it on the lowest setting. When you're finished, strain off the leaf material through a fine mesh strainer. It's definitely not the best way to do it, though. Having leaf and bud to juice is like having gold. You want to make sure you are extracting the maximum amount of nutrients from that plant matter.

Step 1

Picking leaves from the plant well into the flowering stage is ideal but any leaf has benefits. Always juice your leaf as soon as possible for best results. If you cannot juice it right away, keep it fresh in Debbie Meyer Green Bags inside your refrigerator. Do not wash the leaf first.

How many leaves does it take to make a daily dose? That can vary quite a bit, depending on what is the right dose for you and on how large the leaves are. But to give you an example, I weighed it one time and about 1/3 of a pound of fresh leaves without stems and bud yielded about 6 ounces of juice.

Step 2

Remove the thick, coarse center stem and any leaves that look brown or yellow. I haven't tried this yet, but I've heard some people steep the coarse stems and the roots of the plant (after dirt has been removed) in hot water to make a tea.

Step 3

Soak the leaves in cold water for about 10 minutes right before you're ready to juice. The intention here, I believe, is to open up the pores and allow more juice to be extracted. But I'm not really sure. In any case, it does work better to soak it in water first as you can extract more green juice.

Step 4

If you grew the plants yourself, then keep the buds and juice them, too, if the trichomes are fully present and milky but not amber in color. Trichomes are the sticky little hairs on the bud of the cannabis plant.

I spoke with some folks at Resin Seeds about when is the best time to harvest the bud in order to get the maximum amount of CBD. They indicated that CBD seems to be produced before the THC. Therefore if you want lower THC and higher CBD, perhaps harvesting earlier will help since the THC wont become fully developed.

The buds contain significant concentrated amounts of CBD, THC, and other cannabinoids. If you obtained the buds from someone else, I recommend that you find out for certain whether or not the buds became heated. If you're satisfied that they have not been heated then it will be very beneficial for you to juice them.

Ideally, add the juice from two raw unheated buds in with the leaf juice each day. Don't soak the buds in water first because of the crystals on them. Since there's a lot of cannabinoids in those crystals, they may come off in the water.

Buds contain a high concentration of cannabinoids and therefore are very powerful, even if you're only juicing a high THC strain. I have noticed a significant difference between drinking just leaf juice versus drinking bud juice or bud and leaf juice combined. I only need 1 to 3 ice cubes of bud juice to feel improvement. For me the improvement wasn't noticeable immediately but rather a couple of days later. But every one of us is different in that regard.

Step 5
Put the soaked leaves and fresh buds (if you have them) into the Vitamix with a few ice cubes. You'll have to play around with the amount of ice to add, but the ice is necessary to keep the Vitamix from turning your cannabis into a paste versus a fiber-laden juice.

Step 6
Mix it with something fatty such as yogurt, kefir, hemp oil, coconut milk, ice cream, etc., for optimal absorption. The terpenes are fat soluble. I usually make a smoothie by mixing the juice with yogurt and frozen fruit in the Vitamix or other blender.

During a phone consultation, Dr. Courtney advised me not to drink the juice with vegetable or fruit juice, because this would leave behind too much of the beneficial terpenes on the sides of the glass. As mentioned above, always mix the juice with something fatty.

It is best to consume your juice right away. But you can store it in a tightly sealed glass container (before mixing it with other ingredients) for up to 3 days in a refrigerator. Drink it throughout the day in roughly 4 to 6 or more divided doses. If you keep it in the refrigerator for longer than three days, it tastes similar to how orange juice tastes after it's been refrigerated too long. It has a sharp tangy taste to it. I don't know what, if anything, this implies regarding any changes in its efficacy as a medicine but it does not taste good at this point. So, keep it refrigerated for no more than three days and then freeze it or mix it in a smoothie and drink it.

It's easiest to pour the juice into BPA-free ice cube trays with lids or regular ice cube trays and place those trays into sealed Ziploc bags or turkey bags. By sealing the juice you protect the delicate terpenes from getting destroyed. They play a part in the healing process and give the plant its distinct aroma.

And don't make the mistake I did by pouring my juice into ice cube trays of varying sizes. You really should be keeping a daily diary or log of your healing progress with juice and the only way to do that is to know exactly how much juice you are consuming. So count your cubes.

One thing you may consider trying from time to time, once you've achieved some level of healing from drinking cannabis juice, is to lower your dose of juice for a few days up to a week. Then slowly bring your dose back up again. This may reset your endocannabinoid receptors, allowing you to get a greater benefit from less juice. As far as I know this is just anecdotal evidence when it comes to the acidic cannabinoids. But I do know from first-hand experience that with the "neutral" or "active" cannabinoids as they are called (i.e. THC and CBD), that it works very well to take a little break for a few days from consuming them.

Then when you resume you need much less to achieve an effect. But slowly your receptors saturate again and you need more of the medicine to achieve the same result.

Dr. Courtney advised me to drink the juice for the rest of my life in order to achieve the possibility of putting my disease into a long-term remission and keeping it there. To me, this was daunting at first. But once you begin to feel the healing effects of this amazing plant, you know that you will always do your very best to find a way to make sure you have cannabis juice. Since no two people are exactly alike, and there is much more research that needs to be done on cannabis, it's possible that your experience may be different. You may heal completely and never need cannabis again. But as Dr. Courtney puts it, raw cannabis is a "dietary essential." It is considered a vegetable. So even if you're not sick, you may wish to consume raw cannabis because it's extremely health supportive.

Some effects, according to Dr. Courtney, "take three days to be appreciated. Others build for weeks. Full clinical benefit may take 4 to 8 weeks to take effect. It takes that long for plant (phyto) cannabinoids to fully saturate the body's adipose (fat) tissue. Phytocannabinoids are stored in the adipose tissue, as are the fat-soluble vitamins A, D, E, and K."
(http://www.alternet.org/personal-health/juicing-raw-cannabis-miracle-health-cure-some-its-proponents-believe-it-be)

Another option to juicing your cannabis is to just eat it raw. I just started growing some high CBD plants from seed a few weeks ago, and I decided to pick off a few leaves and taste them. They were actually pretty good! I could see eating them in a salad or mixing them into a salsa or pesto sauce. They were slightly spicy tasting. The best part for me was that each time I do this, I feel even better the next day. Probably partly because I'm eating them fresh from the plant therefore I'm receiving all of the plant's vital energy. But I suspect that I mostly feel the benefits from eating the raw leaves from these high CBD plants because of the very fact that they are high in CBD. I have never had the chance to juice high CBD plants. I find it amazing that I have healed this far by only consuming random high THC leaves and bud.

Chapter 10
Cannabis Oil, Tincture & Salve

If you aren't yet at the point where you are able to juice yet or if you are juicing but haven't seen the results you need, you may wish to consider ingesting cannabis-infused olive oil. If you are tired of taking pain medications and/or seeing adverse results from doing so, consider using another part of the plant to manage your pain: The bud. You can smoke or vaporize it, of course, for quick pain relief. But if you don't like inhaling, why not try edibles?

I was completely opposed to edibles at first. They take a while to enter your bloodstream and therefore titration can be difficult at the outset. You can consume too much of a cookie and not know it until an hour or hour and a half later when you recognize that you're outrageously high. It can be a pretty scary feeling. Large doses can cause hallucinations in some people but only trigger sleep in others.

But the good news is that there is a way to eat cannabis moderately. I found that consuming baked goods was difficult because the results varied from cookie to cookie. Instead, consider taking a tiny medicine measuring cup, one that measures in milliliters or teaspoons and fill it with cannabis oil using an eye dropper. Start off very slowly with the smallest measurement possible. Then take a small cup of applesauce and pour the cannabis oil into the applesauce and mix it to make it more palatable.

It can take from maybe 30 minutes to a couple of hours to notice the effects. I notice that it seems to take longer to feel the effects if I consume it on a full stomach. If you don't experience much or any pain relief or a sense of feeling high, then try again the next night with a slightly larger dose. The key word is "slightly." Once you get the dose that's perfect for you, it's fairly safe to say that as long as you are using the same batch of oil, you should get about the same results day after day.

I preferred to use the oil only in the evening because I didn't like the high feeling during the day while I needed to function and go to work, take care of the kids, etc. So I would take it at around 6 p.m. when the pain really kicked in and then I would feel the results around 7 or 7:30 p.m. when it was time to put the kids to bed. It really relaxed my body enough for me to flop on the couch with less pain. But I was never able to tolerate the head high enough to really bring my dose up to the level of obliterating the pain entirely.

Making the oil is easy. Take a crock-pot and fill it with olive oil. Next, submerge a generous portion of dried bud into the oil and set the temperature to the lowest possible setting. Stir it once a day and by the third day it's ready to strain off the plant material through a fine mesh sieve. Pour the oil into glass jars with a tight lid and keep it in a cool, dark place up high, way out of the reach of children.

How much oil and how much bud you use depends on how much you have available. I am unaware of a set or recommended recipe. And how strong your oil is each time you make it will vary widely. That's why I say to go slow and test it little by little. And, of course, don't assume that each batch will be the same. Test it each time to see how much you can tolerate. I used an eye dropper to transfer the oil from the jar into the small measuring cup.

If you consume the oil on a daily basis, you will find that eventually you will need to increase your dosage as your cannabinoid receptors get used to it. You can increase your dose or you can just stop using the oil for a little while to allow the receptors to "reset" themselves. It's interesting to note that the amount of cannabis-infused oil you need to consume to feel the effects has nothing to do with how small or large you are. You build up a tolerance over time and some people seem to have a naturally high tolerance.

There is new anecdotal evidence that eating a mango an hour before you medicate with cannabis will help to lengthen and intensify the euphoric high feeling and the pain-relieving effect. There are a few other edible plants, such as hops, that fall into the same category. You can read a short article about it here http://www.alternet.org/food/mangoes-boost-marijuana-high. This is worth noting in case you notice different effects from day to day without having changed the amount of cannabis oil (or smoke or vapor) that you consumed. It could be due to what you ate an hour earlier.

Another way to manage your pain naturally is by using a tincture. Cannabis tinctures have been around for a very long time—well before the prohibition began. The nice thing about a tincture is that it will give you relatively rapid relief. It should take about 15 minutes for you to feel the effects. They usually come in either an alcohol or glycerin base. Alcohol is generally more effective but it can tend to burn the mouth whereas glycerin is sweeter. You just put a few drops (not droppers) of the tincture under your tongue, swish it around your mouth a bit and wait about 2 to 3 minutes before swallowing. This allows it to do something called "first-pass metabolism." Basically it bypasses your digestive tract and goes straight into your blood stream.

My experience with tinctures (and the experience of some of my friends with tinctures) is that they are very weak. I find edibles to be much more effective, but they do take a lot longer to hit you. But I think I've finally discovered the reason why the tinctures I've tried have been so weak. It's not enough to just dry out the kief (https://www.leafly.com/news/cannabis-101/what-is-kief-anyway), bud, or trim (leftover leaves that you trim off of a bud after harvest)—it needs to be decarboxylated first. So you need to bake it for an hour in the oven at about 240 degrees F before you put it into alcohol or glycerin. Here is a great article about how to do this: http://www.marijuanagrowershq.com/decarboxylating-cannabis-turning-thca-into-thc/.

I have always gotten my tinctures from caregivers or dispensaries so I have not tried this baking method yet but it makes sense to me. I suspect I've found tinctures to be weak because they were only made with dried out plant matter. Meaning there's some decarboxylated (THC) in there but also a lot of acidic cannabinoids (THCa, CBDa). Since I have not made my own tincture yet, I can't recommend any specific recipes but there are many on the Internet. I have tried both alcohol-based and glycerin-based tinctures and, although the glycerin was pretty sticky and a little hard to get out of the dropper, it was much more pleasant to taste than the stinging alcohol ones. But that's really just a matter of personal preference.

One thing to keep in mind is that there are different strains for different pains. So if you don't get relief from one strain, try a different one. And keep trying until you find one that is right for you. There are three general cannabis species: Indica, sativa, and ruderalis. Sativa strains tend to give you energy and are generally known to be good for anxiety and depression whereas indica strains make you want to rest and sleep on the couch and are great for managing body pain and inflammation. So keep that in mind when selecting a strain.

Cannabis ruderalis originates from central Russia and is not as popular or readily available in most places as indica and sativa strains. These plants flower early and can withstand harsh, cold climates. In any case, just remember to start low and go slow; less is best with cannabis. To learn more about the various cannabis strains and to read reviews, check out http://www.leafly.com.

There is a theory floating around in the juicing community that landrace cannabis strains that are a 1:1 ratio may be the most healing strains. Here is how Leafly.com describes landrace strains:

"Historical documents from around the world, some dating as far back as 2900 B.C., tell us cannabis has lived alongside humans for thousands of years, cultivated for religious and medicinal purposes. Many growers believe the earliest cannabis strains sprouted in the Hindu Kush region of Afghanistan and Pakistan and eventually spread to other areas, including South America, Asia, Jamaica, Africa, and even Russia. We call these indigenous strains *landraces*.

"A landrace refers to a local variety of cannabis that has adapted to the environment of its geographic location. This accounts for genetic variation between landrace strains, which have been crossbred to produce the cannabis variety we see today. Landrace strains are oftentimes named after their native region (e.g., Afghani, Thai, Hawaiian), and traces of these forefather strains are sometimes detectable in the names of their crossbred descendants. A combination of environmental conditions and selective breeding by native populations gave rise to these stable varieties, the forefathers of all modern strains."

So these are the strains that existed in nature before man began tinkering with them by selective cross breeding. Animals and humans have grazed on these varieties for thousands of years. Since whole plant synergy of terpenes, cannabinoids, and other healing molecules within the cannabis plant account for its unparalleled healing capability, it may make sense to turn to these stable varieties for their medicinal properties. Nature knows best.

Here is a list of some landrace strains: Hindu Kush (Afghanistan/Pakistan), Pure Afghan (Afghanistan/Pakistan), Lamb's Bread (Jamaica), Acapulco Gold (Mexico), Durban Poison (Africa), Malawi (Africa), and Panama Red (Central America).

One thing to consider when selecting a strain is to smell it first. If it smells bad to you, it may not be the most healing strain for you. If it smells pleasing to you, it's a sign that this strain may be the best strain for you. The smell is from the terpenes.

When you are taking vaporizer hits, just like with tinctures, it can take up to 15 minutes for you to feel the effects. Therefore it is best to wait 15 minutes between vaporizer hits so that you don't overdo it.

When you are medicating with psychoactive cannabis, you need to keep in mind not to overexert yourself. Not that you even want to as most of the time it will make you relaxed or sleepy. In any case, do not exercise while taking it. After you've been lying down for a while, stand up slowly so you don't get a head rush and pass out. While you may not be planning to run a marathon while medicating with cannabis, you may be asked to help someone lift something heavy or do something that requires physical exertion. Don't do it.

Wait until the medication has worn off before you exert yourself. This is to protect your heart.

There are topical salves you can make or purchase. Often they are made from olive oil and beeswax infused with cannabis. The skin is the largest organ in the body therefore it can be an effective way to get your medicine directly to the parts of your body that hurt. I haven't had a lot of success with them but a lot of people swear by salves. Keep in mind that you do not always have to put the salve right on the place that hurts. You can put it on it, around it, and near it. For example, if your knee hurts, put the salve on your knee but also behind your knee and on the sides. Rub it in gently and wait for it to seep into the painful area.

And lastly, there are cannabis oils that are basically highly concentrated essential oils made from cannabis bud. Rick Simpson Oil (see http://www.phoenixtears.ca), as the high THC essential oil is known, can be made at home using a pound of quality 20% or higher THC dried bud. A pound should make enough to last you about three months. If you don't need that much, you can use less bud and scale the recipe accordingly. Here is an excellent video that I've followed that will show you how to make a small batch of RSO: http://bit.ly/1JujPtb

Or you can purchase the oil from a vendor (see http://www.cannabisoilexchange.com) such as a local caregiver or dispensary. Not all caregivers and dispensaries will offer this and there is some risk of explosion involved in making the oil yourself.

But if you follow directions exactly, you will have no problem. My husband made some Rick Simpson Oil for me which I have been applying to various skin cancer spots on my body. It's been almost three weeks and they are healing nicely. One spot is almost all new skin and another spot has new skin emerging but it gets smelly and pussy every other day, forcing me to change the bandage more often than I normally would.

At first the oil seemed to act like a transdermal patch: The medicine was entering my bloodstream. I could tell this because I had some of the symptoms of being high but without the actual high. Basically it made me sleepy. But now I'm used to it and I don't notice any side effects.

The reason I bring up the Rick Simpson Oil is that it is another very effective cannabis medicine. People are being cured of very serious illnesses by consuming this oil, especially cancer. Be sure to purchase and read Rick's very inexpensive eBook (at http://www.phoenixtears.ca) before attempting to make and consume this medicine. You can also make this medicine using high CBD bud, although I do not have much information about how much success people have had with that. Probably because not many people have tried to make it that way. But if you are averse to getting very high, then that may be the way to go for you because regular high THC Rick Simpson Oil will get you high (at least at first until you get used to it) and presumably a CBD-dominant bud will not—or at least not as high.

People use this oil topically (like I am using it, underneath a bandage to heal skin issues), orally, and rectally in suppositories. For best results, Rick advises putting the oil closest to the area where you have the disease. So, for example, if you have bowel cancer, then suppositories may work best for you.

If you would like to bounce questions off of people who have tried these oils, you can seek out various Facebook groups by searching "cannabis oil" or "Rick Simpson Oil."

Another alternative to Rick Simpson Oil is to make a cannabis extract using a cold (unheated) process. David Mapes of Epsilon Apothecaries has created a free guide to teach anyone in detail how to do this at http://www.epsilonresearch.org/#!free-guide.

Chapter 11
Testimonials

"Basically, I lived for many years with unrecognized and untreated epilepsy after a head injury (that is the very short and not too descriptive story). It got really bad, which prompted me to enter the whole medical world and for about seven years I played pharmaceutical roulette, trying many different drug treatments for seizures. I felt like these drugs, while they reduced some of the incapacitating seizures and pain, flattened my emotional landscape and took me away from my true self.

"I found the least objectionable anti-seizure med and took it faithfully for about five years, with one of the greatest difficulties being simply maintaining health insurance to cover the $888 of monthly prescriptions (eventually I enrolled in a program run by the pharmaceutical company that covered the cost, and patients should be aware that these programs exist.)

"The change happened for me when a friend of mine was diagnosed with breast cancer, and although I lived in an illegal state at the time, I worked through friends of friends to get a connection to cannabis medicine for her from the west coast. I found a person who would send smoothie mix and extracts (all untested, no dosage, just hit or miss) for my friend and I started taking it too.

"Please understand, up to that point I had been inhaling cannabis daily ever since the head injury, to some moderate relief, but not enough to control the seizures which really troubled me. When I began to ingest cannabis orally on a daily basis, I found that I felt better, and after a year and a few months I began to wean off of the anti-seizure meds.

"Eventually, I relocated to California, specifically for cannabis freedom. I got my 215 patient recommendation and had my first acdc high CBD plants growing a month after I got here. I also joined a medical collective, found great resources for education about how to juice raw cannabis from my local dispensary (Arcata's Humboldt Patient Resource Center, where Dr. William Courtney initiated the juice protocol a couple of years ago) and learned from fellow patients how to make my own medicine. Although my health is delicate, I was able to work as a trimmer in the cannabis industry, often bartering for the raw materials for my medicine. (I mention this to encourage other patients that where there's a will there's a way, and not to let money stand in the way of treatment.)

"I now use cannabis as my only anti-seizure med, and not only do I feel it helps me with whole body vitality, it manages my neurological condition in a way that, far from the pharmaceuticals that made me feel disconnected and not myself, actually brings me back to the feeling of my true self. I ingest a variety of high CBD, both raw and psychoactive preparations of cannabis every day, and I thank God for its existence and availability in my life."

- Aurora

California, USA

"I have RA. (I have other health issues also.) I just recently started juicing cannabis (it tastes awful, lol), but I've noticed it helps a ton with inflammation. I've been taking RSO [Rick Simpson Oil] for about two years, and it's been incredibly healing. I've found it isn't affordable because I need a gram or more each day to fully relieve my pain. So I started juicing about 2 weeks ago and I've felt a big improvement! I still need RSO but not nearly as much."

- Anon

"To whom it may concern:

"My name is Judi Smith. I was diagnosed with multiple sclerosis in 1991. My mobility is limited, I get fatigued easily, my muscles are very tight and spasmodic plus I have a problem with edema in my weaker leg. I have also been recently diagnosed with hypothyroidism.

"I started looking into cannabis for my medical issues and I came across Dr William Courtney's raw cannabis juice research in America. His patients found that raw cannabis juice helped enormously with and relieved their autoimmune conditions, as well as cancer.

"It is impossible to obtain raw cannabis juice in the UK. However, during my research I came across raw hemp juice, which is virtually the same thing. I started taking raw hemp juice six weeks ago."

"Hemp juice has had a hugely beneficial effect on my energy levels. I am writing this at 5:30 a.m., feeling wide awake and alert. I used to fall asleep in the afternoons and am finding I rarely need to nap in the day now. My bladder is less reactive, my body seems stronger and my leg is not swelling up so much. The hemp juice has had a cleansing and detoxifying effect. I experienced flu-like symptoms for three days and afterwards there was a remarkable shift in my energy levels. I take my hemp juice in the mornings as I found taking it at night kept me awake.

"I truly believe that raw hemp juice should be available on a long-term basis to anyone with a serious health condition. On a related note, the hemp family, *Cannabis sativa* and *C. indica*, should be recognized as medical plants and deregulated so that people can obtain relief from their medical conditions."

- Judi Smith
Brighton, UK

And here's a brief testimonial from the owner of a golden retriever mix dog who contracted Lyme disease:

"After munching fresh, raw cannabis leaves, her blood work was normal and liver enzymes normal."

- San Diego, CA, USA

"I started drinking hemp juice to improve my overall health. I suffered from a maddening core tiredness, joint pain, various IBS symptoms and strong PMS and perimenopausal symptoms.

"I started drinking hemp juice 8-9 months ago sporadically. Two or 3 months ago I made the commitment to remember to drink it every day. I started with one cube, now I drink 3 cubes daily.

"Since my commitment, I've noticed I'm not experiencing PMS or extreme hormonal changes. I have increased energy that is noticeable on a very deep level. It feels like a deep-seated strength and capability. I've now eliminated wheat and haven't felt tired at all, in any way, for the past month. I did experience a healing crisis when I increased to 3 cubes, but it subsided after 3 or 4 days."

- Lisa

"I have Crohn's going on 11 years. I started taking hemp about 4 months ago. I would take one glass in morning before breakfast with water and one spoon of honey. I would say it tastes a little bit like grass. I would feel much better since I start taking hemp. I wouldn't feel as sick since I started taking hemp, and I have lot more energy."

- Ellen

"I was diagnosed with RA in 2013 with rheumatoid factor above 600. I could barely move. My knees and ankles and arms were in pain, and I was so weak I couldn't brush my own hair.
Because of Kristin Courtney's video LEAF I went on a quest for cannabis leaves. I was given quite large amounts of leaves from a grower, and I put them in smoothies and froze a lot. I grew some high CBD strains but not enough to juice because of the 12 plant limitation here. I began to get better. I also stopped all dairy products and went on the Paddison program for RA which is an alkaline diet.

"The cannabis helped a lot. Helped with the inflammation and the pain. I eat raw bud and leaf when I have it and am currently on a high CBD oil.

"I want to do the cancer protocol of approximately a gram a day for about three months to see how it will help. I never went on the chemo pills they wanted me on. Methotrexate is highly toxic. I had no desire to take those medications.

"I juice when I can, eat raw bud and leaf when I have access, and use oil presently that I make according to Epsilon's formula that Dave Mapes has shared. I'm improved to the point I can do serious exercise and have hopes of full remission soon."

- Lynn Thompson

(Note: When Lynn says "serious exercise," she's not kidding. She regularly kickboxes and does krav maga!)

"For me I notice the most benefits from both smoking flower and I use fresh frozen water and sugar leaves in my smoothies! I also have gastroparesis so I have lots of issues. When I read your struggles with many of the same simple daily tasks, I was like, oh, yes, I know how she feels.

"I also use cannabis topicals & bath products I call it my daily 'soak & toke.' well my gasterial paresis is tolerable now where before I got my mmj prescription I would have flare ups at least every other month! Those consist of non-stop throwing up, horrible stomach pains, loose bowels, etc. The longest bout I had was 2 weeks of not keeping ANYTHING down...not even water!! Both my diseases are autoimmune. I do not use any pharmaceuticals. I don't really measure the leaf amount—maybe ½ cup for a smoothie. My a.m. remedy is dabs for my arthritis and flowers; for my gastro, 2 smoothies or day 1 in a.m. 4 protein, one before bed for anti-inflammatory. And I use both hemp and/or flax meal (not in same smoothie). I only do the fresh or raw juicing in summer when have my outdoor garden."

- Tina Leger

"My name is Debbie Hansen. I'm a 63-year-old grandmother, a veteran's widow and disabled nurse. In 2003 I was diagnosed with stage 3b breast cancer (infiltrating ductal carcinoma). From the getgo I refused conventional treatment (chemotherapy and radiation), although I had repeated surgical interventions leading to double mastectomies. I was told to put my affairs in order and was refused breast reconstruction due to the cancer cells returning. I basically was sent home to die. I also have severe osteoarthritis, severe osteoporosis, fibromyalgia, neuropathy, and neuralgia. I was started on narcotics for pain control and ended up in a narcotic fog for 10 years. Then one day I decided to take my life back. I weaned myself off my narcotics and other pharmaceuticals (20+) and started full extract cannabis oil for the cancer and chronic pain issues. What a miracle! I am now cancer free and the University of Washington did my breast reconstruction and my pathology reports are negative for cancer. I have almost completed my breast reconstruction. Unfortunately, due to the new medical cannabis laws in Washington State and my fixed income, I have been forced back to some pharmaceuticals, which is very distressing to me."

- Debbie Hansen

(Note: Debbie did juice as well from one plant that she grew herself.)

AUTHOR'S UPDATE:

I've been juicing almost every single day now for a year and a half. Sometimes I eat the leaf straight from the plant, too, but not in large quantities. I just nibble as I tend to them. I believe I am close to full remission now. The reason I say that "I believe" I'm close to full remission is because I still have a little pain due to damage done from the RA. But compared to how I felt a year and a half ago, it's minimal. My feet hurt and my right knee has some swelling. My right wrist doesn't fully bend and the middle of my back slightly aches upon waking.

But I have tons of energy and I've pretty much returned to my regular life, except I don't go jogging at the moment. Lately I've been able to do a half hour Spin bike class followed by 20 minutes of modified yoga (no salute to the sun for me yet), and lots of short hikes. I am so incredibly grateful for having found this plant. If I can heal, then most likely you can, too, as I had an extremely severe case of inflammation that was not responding well to traditional or alternative therapies.

Do I expect to always have sore feet and other minor issues? No, I do not. I met a man last year at a publicity summit I attended in New York City who many years ago became a quadriplegic as a result of a major car accident. He almost completely healed himself with qi gong and tai chi. You can read his story in this article in the

Arizona Daily Star: http://bit.ly/1H1MVuP. Can you imagine someone healing a broken back and neck? If that's possible, anything is possible. By the way, if movement is painful for you and the idea of doing even something as gentle as yoga is out of reach at the moment, look into qi gong and tai chi. I did it when I was having a minor flare up this past winter and it really helped to loosen me up and make me feel a better.

My sincere hope is that this book gives you some hope. Hope to heal and return to perfect health. I wish you the very best on your healing journey.

Do you have a testimonial you would like to share? Then please email me at katie@juicingcannabisforhealing.com. If you do not wish to use your name or contact information, please indicate that in the email. This book is like a living, breathing organism in that it will be constantly evolving, being updated with new information and testimonials. Anything we can share with each other will help all of us and future readers who may wish to experience juicing cannabis for healing. Also, please like our Facebook page at http://www.facebook.com/juicingpot to follow the latest medical marijuana and cannabis juicing news.

Appendix A
Links to US States' Laws Regarding Medical Marijuana

I recommend visiting the regulatory licensing body governmental website in your state and read their statute. Then call that government agency and ask the following questions:

1. What diseases are medical marijuana cards issued for in our state? (Or just tell them your issue to see if you will be covered.)

2. Am I allowed to grow my own cannabis for my personal medical use or do I need to purchase my medicine from a dispensary or caregiver?

3. How many plants can I grow or how much usable material (i.e., buds, edibles, tinctures, salves, juice) am I allowed to possess at one time?

4. Is there a difference in the number of mature flowering plants I can have at one time versus immature non-flowering plants?

5. How many seeds and/or seedlings can I have at one time?

6. Where can I grow it? (For example, some states restrict growing cannabis to a locked room indoors or outdoors with a high fence around the plants.)

7. Do I need to obtain a medical marijuana card or prescription from a medical doctor or other medical professional?

8. Where can I obtain a list of licensed doctors or other medical professionals who provide marijuana prescriptions?

9. How long is the card valid and how much does it cost?

10. Does our state have a state registry of patients? Is this information kept confidential?

The following is a list of links to government agencies that regulate the issuing of medical marijuana cards for 23 US states and the District of Columbia. Please research the local laws in your country before you begin your healing journey. For an up-to-date map of the ever-changing cannabis laws in the US, check out NORML's website at http://norml.org/laws/.

Alaska
http://dhss.alaska.gov/dph/VitalStats/Pages/marijuana.aspx

Arizona

http://www.azdhs.gov/medicalmarijuana/index.htm

California

http://www.cdph.ca.gov/programs/mmp/Pages/default.aspx

Colorado

http://1.usa.gov/1hzhs4a

Connecticut

http://1.usa.gov/1rqEx2L

District of Columbia

http://1.usa.gov/UhYOsT

Delaware

http://dhss.delaware.gov/dhss/dph/hsp/medmarhome.html

Hawaii

http://dps.hawaii.gov/about/divisions/law-enforcement-division/ned/

Illinois

http://www.idph.state.il.us/HealthWellness/MedicalCannabis/index.htm

Maine

http://www.maine.gov/dhhs/dlrs/mmm/index.shtml

Maryland
http://1.usa.gov/1tiwqTM

Massachusetts
http://www.mass.gov/eohhs/gov/departments/dph/programs/hcq/medical-marijuana/

Michigan
http://1.usa.gov/1qoRQRK

Minnesota
http://www.health.state.mn.us

Montana
http://www.dphhs.mt.gov/marijuanaprogram/

Nevada
http://health.nv.gov/MedicalMarijuana.htm

New Hampshire
http://www.dhhs.state.nh.us/oos/tcp/index.htm

New Jersey
http://www.state.nj.us/health/medicalmarijuana/

New Mexico

http://nmhealth.org/about/mcp/svcs/

New York

http://www.health.ny.gov/regulations/medical_marijuana/

Oregon

http://www.oregon.gov/oha/mmj/Pages/index.aspx

Rhode Island

http://www.health.ri.gov/programs/medicalmarijuana/

Vermont

http://vcic.vermont.gov/marijuana_registry

Washington

http://1.usa.gov/Wr0L80

Appendix B
List of Seed Banks

Here is a list of cannabis seed banks that you can order from, if you choose to go that route. Some seed banks have websites and offer online ordering; in other cases, you may have to obtain seeds from health centers or dispensaries. Some of the companies are in the US and others are overseas. I have never personally ordered from any of these companies but the first 10 are taken from the *High Times* 2014 list of seed bank hall of famers. In my opinion, *High Times* is a trusted resource of cannabis information. They have been around since 1974. You can read a bit about the history and their review of each seed bank here:

http://www.hightimes.com/read/2014-seed-bank-hall-fame.

La Plata Labs
http://www.laplatalabs.com

Rare Dankness
http://www.raredankness.com

Karma Genetics
http://www.karmagenetics.com

Grand Daddy Purp Genetics

http://www.granddaddypurp.com

Elemental Seeds
http://www.elementalseeds.com

Archive Seed Bank
http://www.archiveseedbank.com

Loud Seeds
http://www.loudseeds.com

Devil's Harvest
http://www.thedevilsharvestseeds.com

Hortilab Seeds
http://www.hortilabseeds.com

MTG Seeds
http://www.mtgseeds.com

List of vendors of CBD-rich seeds:

Resin Seeds
Mail order from Spain
http://www.resinseeds.net

Reggae Seeds
Mail order from Spain

http://www.reggaeseeds.com

CBD Crew

Mail order seeds from Europe

http://www.cbdcrew.org

Appendix C
US States Allowed to Grow Hemp for Research as Per 2014 US Farm Bill

The following is quoted verbatim from the National Conference of State Legislatures (http://www.ncsl.org/research/agriculture-and-rural-development/state-industrial-hemp-statutes.aspx) as of 6/20/2014.

"The final 2014 Farm Bill agreement included a provision that would allow institutions of higher education and state departments of agriculture to grow or cultivate industrial hemp.

"It also requires that the sites used by universities and agriculture department be certified by—and registered with—their state department of agriculture. This provision will allow universities and agricultural departments to study industrial hemp for its possible future use as a commercial product.

"Fifteen states—California, Colorado, Hawaii, Indiana, Kentucky, Maine, Montana, Nebraska, North Dakota, Oregon, South Carolina, Tennessee, Utah, Vermont, and West Virginia—currently have laws to provide for hemp production as described by the

Farm Bill stipulations. Nine of these states—California, Colorado, Maine, Montana, North Dakota, Oregon, Vermont, and West Virginia—sponsored hemp resolutions and have laws to promote the growth and marketing of industrial hemp.

"Current state policies include:
- Defining industrial hemp based on the percentage of tetrahydrocannabinol it contains.
- Authorizing the growing and possessing of industrial hemp.
- Requiring state licensing of industrial hemp growers.
- Promoting research and development of markets for industrial hemp.
- Excluding industrial hemp from the definition of controlled substances under state law.
- Establishing a defense to criminal prosecution under drug possession or cultivation

State Statutes

California

CA FOOD & AG §81000-81010
- Requires industrial hemp growers to be registered with the state.
- Prohibits the possession of resin, flowering tops or leaves removed from the hemp plant.
- Establishes registration and renewal fees for

commercial growers of industrial hemp.
- Organizes a five year review of industrial hemp's economic impact.
- While legislation adding this section was enacted in 2013, the law specifies that its provisions do not become operative unless authorized by federal law.

Colorado

CRS § 25-18.7-101 to -105

- Permits growing and possessing industrial hemp.
- Establishes industrial hemp remediation pilot program 'to determine how soils and water may be made more pristine and healthy by phytoremediation, removal of contaminants, and rejuvenation through the growth of industrial hemp.'

Hawaii

S.B. 2175 (Signed by Governor on April 30, 2014)

- 'Authorizes the dean of the College of Tropical Agriculture and Human Resources at the University of Hawaii at Manoa to establish an industrial hemp remediation and biofuel crop research program;
- requires a report on the rate of contamination uptake and efficient uptake from soil and water, the rate of carbon fixation in the Calvin cycle and the viability of industrial hemp as a biofuel feedstock;
- clarifies that the term industrial hemp means the

plant *Cannabis sativa* L.;
- provides criminal and civil immunity.'

Indiana
IC 15-15-13-7

- 'Industrial hemp is an agricultural product that is subject to regulation by the state seed commissioner.'
- The state seed commissioner adopts rules and oversees licensing, production, and management of industrial hemp and agricultural hemp seed.
- Sets the standards for application for hemp license and registration.

Kentucky
KRS § 260.850-.869

- Establishes research on industrial hemp and industrial hemp products.
- 'Industrial hemp means all parts and varieties of the plant *Cannabis sativa*, cultivated or possessed by a licensed grower, whether growing or not, that contain a tetrahydrocannabinol concentration of one percent (1%) or less by weight, except that the THC concentration limit of one percent (1%) may be exceeded for licensed industrial hemp seed research.
- 'The Department of Agriculture shall promote the research and development of markets for Kentucky

industrial hemp and hemp products after the selection and establishment of the industrial hemp research program and the Industrial Hemp Commission…'

- Includes language that 'Kentucky shall adopt the federal rules and regulations that are currently enacted regarding industrial hemp and any subsequent changes thereto.'
- On Feb. 19, 2014, Kentucky announced five pilot hemp projects that would be used across the state, including one project that would research whether industrial hemp could be used to remediate tainted soil.

Maine

7 M.R.S.A. § 2231

- Requires industrial hemp growers be licensed by the state.
- Permits a person to 'plant, grow, harvest, possess, process, sell and buy industrial hemp' if that person holds a license.
- Prohibits the state from issuing a license unless 'The United States Congress excludes industrial hemp from the definition of "marihuana" for the purpose of the Controlled Substances Act, 21 United States Code, Section 802(16); or…the United States Department of Justice, Drug Enforcement Administration takes affirmative steps

towards issuing a permit under 21 United States Code, Chapter 13, Subchapter 1, Part C to a person holding a license issued by a state to grow industrial hemp.'

17-A M.R.S. § 1101-1117

- Under criminal code, it is an affirmative defense to drug trafficking, furnishing, cultivation or possession charges if the substance so used is industrial hemp.
- 'Industrial hemp means any variety of *Cannabis sativa L.* with a delta-9- tetrahydrocannabinol concentration that does not exceed 0.3% on a dry weight basis and that is grown under a federal permit in compliance with the conditions of that permit.'

Montana

Mont. Code Anno., § 80-18-101 to 80-18-111

- States that industrial hemp that does not contain more than 0.3% tetrahydrocannabinol is an agricultural product.
- '...an individual in this state may plant, grow, harvest, possess, process, sell, or buy industrial hemp if the industrial hemp does not contain more than 0.3% tetrahydrocannabinol.'
- Requires industrial hemp growers be licensed by the state.

- Creates an affirmative defense to prosecution under criminal code for marijuana possession or cultivation.

Nebraska

NE L 101 (signed by governor on April 2, 2014)

- 'To permit growth and cultivation of industrial hemp by a postsecondary institution or the Department of Agriculture as prescribed
- To exempt industrial hemp from the Uniform Controlled Substances Act as prescribed
- To provide powers and duties for the Department of Agriculture
- And to repeal the original section.

North Dakota

N.D. Cent. Code, § 4-41-01 to 4-41-03 (2009)

- States that industrial hemp that does not contain more than 0.3% is considered an oilseed.
- '…any person in this state may plant, grow, harvest, possess, process, sell, and buy industrial hemp (*Cannabis sativa L.*) having no more than three-tenths of one percent tetrahydrocannabinol.'
- Requires industrial hemp growers be licensed by the state.
- 'North Dakota state university [sic] and any other person licensed under this chapter may import and resell industrial hemp seed that has been certified as

having no more than three-tenths of one percent tetrahydrocannabinol.'

Oregon

O.R.S. § 475.005

- Excludes industrial hemp from definition of 'controlled substance.'

O.R.S. § 571.300 to .315

- Requires industrial hemp growers be licensed by the state.
- Authorizes 'industrial hemp production and possession, and commerce in industrial hemp commodities and products.'

South Carolina

S. 839 (Enacted on June 12, 2014; awaiting Governor's signature)

- 'Adds chapter 55 concerning industrial hemp; provides that it is lawful to grow industrial hemp in this state;
- clarifies that industrial hemp is excluded from the definition of marijuana;
- prohibits growing industrial hemp and marijuana on the same property or otherwise growing marijuana in close proximity to industrial hemp to disguise the marijuana growth.'

Tennessee

TN AG Code 916 (Enacted on May 13, 2014)

- 'Authorizes growing of industrial hemp subject to regulation by the Department of Agriculture;
- provides for license fees;
- provides that industrial hemp is not marijuana but can be categorized as a controlled substance under specified circumstances;
- provides that the department has the right to inspect the hemp crop for compliance.'

Utah

UT H 105 (enacted March 20, 2014)

- Permits the Department of Agriculture and a certified higher education institution to grow industrial hemp for education.
- Exempts an individual with intractable epilepsy who uses or possesses hemp extract or an individual who administers hemp extract to a minor with intractable epilepsy.
- Provides for a hemp extract registration card; requires maintenance of neurologist medical records and a database of neurologist evaluations.

Vermont

6 V.S.A. § 561 to 566

- 'Industrial hemp means varieties of the plant *Cannabis sativa* having no more than 0.3 percent tetrahydrocannabinol, whether growing or not, that are cultivated or possessed by a licensed grower in

- compliance with this chapter.'
- 'Industrial hemp is an agricultural product which may be grown, produced, possessed, and commercially traded in Vermont …'
- Requires industrial hemp growers to be licensed by the state.

West Virginia

W. Va. Code § 19-12E-1 to 19-12E-9

- 'Industrial hemp that has not more than one percent tetrahydrocannabinol is considered an agricultural crop in this state if grown for…purposes authorized…'
- Requires industrial hemp growers be licensed by the state.
- Creates a complete defense to prosecution under criminal code for marijuana possession or cultivation."

Appendix D
Links to US Congress
Listed by State and District

If, by now, you wish to try juicing, then I strongly urge you to take action. Please click the three links below and find your US Representative and Senators and contact The White House. Either call them or feel free to cut and paste the letter at the bottom of this page adapted and expanded from the political action group NORML's website (http://www.norml.org). This letter urges your congressional representatives and the President to end the federal prohibition on marijuana and expand the number of plants allowed to accommodate juicing. There are more moderate measures being introduced via the NORML website, but I figure you should ask for what you really want instead of just baby steps. Because if enough of us ask, we may just get what we need!

I plan to spread the word far and wide via this book and by speaking on radio shows around the US and possibly elsewhere. If we all take action, I truly believe we will eventually see results. The wave of social change regarding medical cannabis has already begun. We just have to ride it to the shore.

Contact Your Representative Here:
http://www.house.gov/representatives/

Contact Your Senators Here:

http://www.senate.gov/general/contact_information/senators_cfm.cfm

Contact President and First Lady Obama Here:

http://www.whitehouse.gov/contact/submit-questions-and-comments

End Federal Marijuana Prohibition and Expand Number of Plants Allowed to Accommodate Juicing for Healing Disease

Never in modern history has there existed greater public support for ending the nation's nearly century-long experiment with marijuana prohibition and replacing it with regulation. The historic votes on Election Day in Colorado and Washington—where, for the first time ever, a majority of voters decided at the ballot box to abolish cannabis prohibition—underscore this political reality.

The ongoing enforcement of cannabis prohibition financially burdens taxpayers, encroaches upon civil liberties, engenders disrespect for the law, impedes legitimate scientific research into the plant's medicinal properties, and disproportionately impacts communities of color.

A majority of voters support regulating the adult consumption of cannabis, according to a variety of national polls. Further, according to a December 2012 Gallup poll, 64 percent of respondents do not believe that the federal government "should take steps to enforce federal anti-marijuana laws in those states" that have legalized the plant.

It is time to stop ceding control of the marijuana market to untaxed criminal enterprises and it is time for lawmakers to impose common-sense regulations governing cannabis and licensing its production. A pragmatic regulatory framework that allows for limited licensed production, sale, and taxation of cannabis best reduces the risks associated with its use or abuse. I encourage you to support legislation to regulate marijuana, not criminalize it.

Furthermore, there is a growing movement among medical cannabis consumers who are juicing the unheated leaves and bud of the cannabis plant in order to alleviate pain and suffering and, in many cases, achieve long-term sustained remission from such diseases. **The unheated plant is non-psychoactive**.

The number of plants needed to produce such juice is substantial. I urge you to make the humane decision to expand the number of plants patients are allowed to grow in states permitting cannabis for medical purposes and extend this to future federal laws. Please view the video on the home page of http://www.cannabisinternational.org and read *Juicing Cannabis for Healing* http://www.amazon.com/dp/B00LWCY196 to learn more.

Thank you for your time and compassion.

Other Books by Katie Marsh

Embracing Quincy
Our Journey Together

What happens when you're told your baby will not live? And if by some miracle she does live, she will be extremely disabled? When a high-tech ultrasound at 22 weeks revealed that Quincy may have a rare genetic disorder called trisomy 18, the Marsh family was given a choice: to terminate or to continue **Embracing Quincy**.

Embracing Quincy takes you on the path almost never traveled by a couple that is decidedly not religious but very spiritually oriented. It shows you a naked glimpse into their personal lives, their travels and their mystical journey with their trisomy 18 baby Quincy.

Embracing Quincy is full of stories of love, humor, psychic phenomena and mystical coincidences that will make even the most skeptical start to question their beliefs. This book will take you to far away lands as it weaves Quincy's story in and out of the Marsh's moves and travels and search for creating a sustainable farm on which to raise their family.

This book non-judgmentally explores issues such as "pro life" versus "pro choice" abortion decisions, karma and reincarnation, the possibility of effecting miracles through quantum physics and the law of attraction, and the power of prayer in large numbers.

Most of all, *Embracing Quincy* shows what a mother and father will do for the love of their unborn baby.

The Birth of Dying
Explore End-of-Life Issues with Your Terminally Ill or Elderly Loved One

by

Katie & Dan Marsh

Are you looking for a way to communicate with your loved one about end-of-life issues?

Fear of pain, fear of the unknown, fear of being forgotten. Wanting to be remembered, wanting to be heard, wanting to be known and truly understood. Is there an afterlife? Who created us, if anyone, and how do I perceive him or her to be? These are some of the basic human issues that connect us all. They are explored here in detail. There are no answers in this workbook—only questions. The right questions. You provide the answers that are right for you.

This workbook addresses most of the concerns and questions we all have about aging and dying. Death can be a taboo topic in our society but an important one to address. Whether you are young and healthy wanting to be prepared for the future or if you are facing terminal illness or hospice, this workbook is a powerful tool that will assist you in communication about aging and eldercare.

The Birth of Dying is designed to be worked through by two people together: daughter to parent, husband to wife, friend to friend, loved one to loved one. Or it can be completed as a private journey of reflection by one person.

The Birth of Dying will help you:

- Explore your thoughts and feelings about your life and your beliefs about religion, spirituality, death, and the possibility of an afterlife
- Share any fears you may have about terminal illness, hospice, and the end-of-life transition
- Prepare an advance directive
- Plan your funeral and leave exact directions for its execution
- Leave a last will and testament for your family in order to bequeath your possessions and direct who shall care for your loved ones after you die
- Write a memoir for your friends and family to remember you by. The back of the workbook contains a detailed template containing questions to help you write a memoir.

Fill it in and leave it for your family to cherish or use it as a launching point for writing your full memoirs.

Whether you or a loved one is facing hospice or a terminal illness, death can be a difficult topic to broach. Communication about aging and eldercare is essential at this stage of life. *The Birth of Dying* is the tool you need to bridge the communication gap.

The Parenting Game Plan
Negotiate, Compromise and Explore the Parenting Journey Together

Have you ever wished you could read someone's mind? Especially your spouse's mind? Although it may not be possible to become a mind reader overnight, you can know your partner's thoughts and feelings about all aspects of child rearing -- *even before the birth of your first child*. This workbook promises to:

- Deliver many example parenting scenarios from before birth through the teenage years for you to think about and discuss with your spouse
- Stimulate your creative juices in coming up with your own compromises and solutions as a couple, thus preventing many possible future disagreements
- Procure examples of how couples with different parenting styles have handled each child raising scenario

- Help you feel closer as a couple as you come up with the answers that are right for your family

We don't need experts telling us how to raise our children in a one-size-fits-all manner. We have all the answers we need inside each of us. We just need the right questions to bring forth the answers that are right for us.

And when you're raising kids, you become a planner. You have to in order to stay one step ahead of the kids. And as a planner, you wouldn't embark on a long road trip without mapping your route. This book is a must-have for the most important journey you and your partner will ever make: Parenthood.

How to Emotionally Heal from Miscarriage, Stillbirth or Early Infant Loss

Did you know about one in four pregnancies ends in miscarriage? My name is Katie Marsh and I have had three miscarriages plus my daughter Quincy who was born at 33 weeks in 2012 and lived just five days. I've also been blessed with two beautiful daughters, ages 5 and 7.

I know loss. I know how much it hurts and I also know that you can get through it and become a happy person again. But of course you never forget the experience and you never forget your baby.

So many of us shove away painful experiences and look in the other direction. We wish we could just run away from ourselves. But sometimes, if we're brave enough, and when we're ready, we can look at the unthinkable straight on and grow. Grow emotionally, spiritually and be more of who we truly are. My hope is that this small yet powerful booklet will help you heal emotionally so you can not just return to your normal life but become even stronger for the experience.

You can purchase these books on amazon.com or on our website at http://www.juicingcannabisforhealing.com/books.html.

To give you a taste of the book I've written that is closest to my heart and that I am most proud of, please enjoy the first chapter of *Embracing Quincy, Our Journey Together*.

The Kick

In silence we drove the five miles from the high-tech ultrasound office to Dan's parents' beach house to pick up the girls. We tried to act like everything was okay but it had been about five hours since we had dropped them off, so his parents looked worried.

"Everything okay?" his mom asked.

"No," I smiled, fighting back the tears. We gave her a brief version of what the doctor told us, then hurriedly packed up the truck with the girls and their many stuffed animals and sundries so we could make the hour-and-a-half trek back up the mountains to Julian before dark.

Thankfully, on the way home the girls fell asleep in the back of our pickup. It was a Ford F-250 that we bought a couple of weeks earlier so that we'd have enough room for three car seats in the roomy back seat yet still have enough utility to pick up hay for Dan's horse and make the rutted off-road journey through the mountain pass to reach our gold claim on the weekends.

"What do you think about this? Is he right?" I asked Dan.

"The equipment was pretty high tech. But it's an ultrasound; it's never foolproof. The amnio will tell us more," Dan tried to reassure me.

"Yeah, but it has its dangers. What if they poke her in the eye with the needle?" I paused for a while, still in major shock. I desperately felt like I wanted to run away from this problem but knew that I couldn't. Quincy and I were attached physically, emotionally and spiritually.

"What do you think about what the doctor said about 'some parents would terminate'?" I questioned Dan, testing the waters to gauge if we had the same thoughts about this subject. "I'm 22 weeks. I *feel* her moving inside of me."

At that exact moment I felt Quincy kick. And she kicked very hard—like never before. *And never afterwards.* She moved and kicked and thrashed around, so much so that I started to fret that she was in some kind of physical distress. Was the cord strangling her suddenly?

"Whoa," I exclaimed as I clutched my belly with both hands, startled and a bit frightened by the sudden violent movement. After a moment I sensed that she wasn't in physical danger. "Dan, feel this!" I whispered, trying not to wake up the kids. He removed his right hand from the steering wheel and allowed me to guide it to the correct spot on my belly.

Wide-eyed, I turned awkwardly in my seat to face Dan. "She *hears* me. She *knows* what I'm saying!"

About the Author

Katie Marsh is an indie author, wife, and mother of two. With health and fitness as lifelong passions, she spent time as an Ironman triathlete and attended a vegetarian cooking school in NYC. She worked many years as a freelance court reporter and as a stenographer for the US House of Representatives. Bored and looking for adventure, she took off backpacking part of the world, spending time in Thailand, Cambodia, Australia, and Hawaii. After a long bout with severe, crippling rheumatoid arthritis, she discovered a natural cure by drinking daily cannabis juice smoothies. As a result, she's become a passionate medical marijuana activist, speaking on radio shows around the US. Today she lives with her family and many critters on a 25-acre burgeoning sustainable farm in Northern Maine.

Made in the USA
San Bernardino, CA
08 April 2016